Making Babies

THE HOLISTIC
IVF
DIET GUIDE

Making Babies

THE HOLISTIC
IVF
DIET GUIDE

Naturopath & Fertility Expert
JENNY BLONDEL
MRN. ND. Dip Nut. Dip BM. Dip Hom. Dip RM.

DAISA & CO
Est. 2003

First published in Great Britain in 2019 by Daisa & Co

A CIP catalogue record for this book is available from the British Library.

ISBN 978-1-9164928-5-1

Book typeset by:
DAISA & CO
Westfield Lakes, Far Ings Road, Barton upon Humber
North Lincolnshire, DN18 5RG, England
www.daisa-co.com

Printed and bound by CPI Group (UK) Ltd, Croydon, CR0 4YY

MIX
Paper | Supporting responsible forestry
FSC® C013604

Daisa & Co is committed to a sustainable future for our business, our readers and our planet. This book in your hands is made from paper certified by the forest stewardship council.

Dedication

This book is dedicated to my best friend and husband...
For his support on our own IVF journey and his unrelenting patience whilst I wrote this book!

To our beautiful IVF miracle boys, Felix and Sebastian...
How immensely blessed we are!

About the Author

Jenny Blondel is a registered naturopath, nutritionist, homoeopath and medical herbalist, and a fertility expert. She is the author of the popular '*The Natural PCOS Diet*'.

Jenny is a member of the:

- British Naturopathic Association (BNA)
- General Council and Register of Naturopaths (GCRN)
- Australian Traditional Medical Society (ATMS).

With 25 years' experience in clinical practice, Jenny is passionate about women's health, fertility and the quest to bring healthy babies into the world. One of the greatest satisfactions of her work is when patients tell her they are finally pregnant.

Jenny was born in Sydney, Australia and lived there at least half of her life and the other half either living in sunny Queensland or in picturesque Yorkshire, England. She is a wife, a mum, a sister and a daughter.

She loves healthy food, cooking and is an enthusiastic Thermomix user. In her spare time, Jenny loves to do yoga, read books, go walking and catch up with friends over a cup of tea.

Keep in Touch

Please visit jennyblondel.com to sign up for Jenny's IVF newsletter, filled with advice, research news, recipes and health tips. You can follow her on Facebook at 'JennyBlondelNaturopath', Twitter at 'IVFdiet' and Instagram jenny.blondel.

In Clinic

You are welcome to contact her to arrange an in-person or online consultation at a convenient time.

For more information about this book and Jenny Blondel visit: jennyblondel.com

Contents

Preface

It is worrying to know how far-reaching and widespread fertility issues have become. It's now estimated that about one in six couples struggle to conceive. In recent years, I have seen a significant increase in patients at my clinic seeking to improve their chances of conceiving, whether it is naturally or with the help of IVF. Having been on the IVF rollercoaster, I know the joy it can bring and the heartache too.

For my husband and me, IVF was our only option to assist us in becoming parents. And it worked! We have two beautiful IVF-conceived boys.

As a result, I want to share my professional expertise and personal experience to provide you with the best and most up-to-date information on diet, functional nutritional medicine, fertility herbs, acupuncture and other treatments to help you look after yourself physically and emotionally in a holistic way.

In my book, I share with you steps you can take to support and prepare for your IVF journey and give you the best possible chance of IVF success.

The birth of a little IVF baby makes me so happy. I feel really proud that I have been able to help bring a new life into this world.

So, let's get started!

Yours in health,

Jenny Blondel

MRN. ND. Dip Nut. Dip BM. Dip Hom. Dip RM.
Naturopath and Fertility Expert

Introduction

It's a myth that relaxing or 'giving it time' will overcome infertility. Fertility problems are frequently medical in nature and can often be treated.

There are over 3 million IVF babies in the world, and we want more! With the right approach, the results speak for themselves.

There is an epidemic of infertility, and in many cases, doctors do not know all the answers. Nor do we naturopaths and other complementary health practitioners. But we all have a common goal – to assist you in becoming pregnant in the hope of delivering a beautiful healthy baby into the world.

The purpose of this book is to encourage you to restore optimal health on all levels through simple naturopathic strategies. This will help ensure you are in the best state of health physically, mentally and emotionally for your IVF journey.

How can this book help you?

For many years I have been treating women and couples with fertility problems, including naturopathic adjunct support for IVF. I know from firsthand experience what it takes to get results, and I want to share my practical advice with you. Imagine having all the information you need from an expert to maximise your chances of IVF. This book is my step-by-step guide to help you on your quest to have a healthy baby.

Making Babies: The Holistic IVF Diet Guide will help you understand:

- How to improve egg quality and the uterine lining to encourage healthy and viable conception

- How to manage your immune system's response to embryo implantation
- How to provide the essential antioxidant support to prevent damage to sperm and egg
- The latest research and nutritional treatments that can be safely and effectively taken with IVF injections and medications
- The best foods to help follicle growth, improve egg quality and strengthen the uterine lining
- The most up-to-date preconception and lifestyle advice
- How to maximise sperm health with a free dedicated book on male reproductive health
- How to remain 'sane' during the two-week wait after embryo transfer with highly effective visualisation techniques, flower essences and more.

In vitro fertilisation (IVF) is probably the most well-known type of assisted reproductive technology (ART) treatment, hence the name of my book. However, there are several other types of ART treatments, including:

- Intrauterine insemination (IUI)
- Frozen Embryo Transfer (FET)
- In Vitro Maturation (IVM)
- Gamete Intrafallopian Transfer (GIFT)
- Zygote Intrafallopian Transfer (ZIFT)
- Intracytoplasmic Sperm Injection (ICSI) for men.

Although I mainly refer to IVF, the recommendations in this book are just as relevant for all the above technologies. The term 'IVF' used in this book covers all the other types of ART.

The term 'doctor' used in this book covers all doctors and specialists involved in IVF, including reproductive endocrinologists, IVF specialists, IVF consultants, gynaecologists and obstetricians.

For my single mums-to-be and couples needing to use donor sperm, I have been sensitive to this issue and have included the men's guide as a bonus/appendix, rather than being included in this book. There is also very relevant information in this book for couples who need to use donor eggs.

How to use this book

There is a great deal of information that can help you maximise your chances of IVF success. This book presents the information in an easy-to-understand form so you can implement the recommendations yourself (I say most as I do recommend you also seek guidance from a qualified naturopath for specific advice and other complementary practitioners such as acupuncturists).

By following the recommendations in this book, you will give yourself the best possible chance of IVF success by improving your general health as well as the quality of your eggs and sperm health for men. As a bonus, you will hopefully feel better, fitter and more energetic.

As you read the recommendations, you'll realise that the changes you make to increase your chance of IVF success are the same as those that will help protect you from miscarriage and produce a healthy baby.

Doctors and IVF consultants are busy people and, all too often, over-worked. The minute you come out of the consulting room you think of a dozen more questions you wanted to ask and discuss. There just isn't time to talk in as much depth as you would like. Yet you want to find out as much as possible. This book is designed to answer many of those questions you may have as well as present a comprehensive self-help programme that will give you and your partner the best chance of conceiving using IVF.

- Section 1 - explains the causes of infertility; what tests are available to help identify such causes; the ins and out of IVF treatment; and where naturopathic support fits in.
- Section 2 - explains how you can help improve your fertility, concentrating on a three-step IVF preconception preparation plan that focuses on gentle detoxification, good nutrition and supplementing your diet. This is one of the most crucial sections of the book as it could be the key to maximising IVF success.
- Section 3 – explains obstacles to overcome, including stress, weight gain, thyroid gland problems, inflammation, elevated homocysteine, MTHFR gene mutations, immune problems, clotting disorders and luteal phase defect.
- Section 4 – provides an in-depth guide to the most suitable diet to follow for IVF – the nitty gritty of the book!
- Section 5 – discusses the best nutritional supplements to use for each phase of the IVF process.
- Section 6 – explains the role of acupuncture, healthy lifestyle choices, massage, relationship support, flower essences and bioresonance.
- Section 7 – provides advice on how to survive the two-week wait following embryo transfer using breathing techniques, meditation and visualisation.
- Section 8 – discusses the problems of implantation failure and miscarriage, and how to deal with these devastating outcomes.
- Section 9 - tells how to care for yourself in pregnancy to maximise your chance of having a healthy baby.

Like your doctor, I make no claims or promises that by following such recommendations you will become pregnant and go on to have a healthy baby.

My aim is to get you and your partner into optimal health using the recommendations outlined in this book, giving you the best possible chance of having your much longed-for, healthy baby.

I believe that any couple planning to have a baby would benefit from following the recommendations outlined in this book, not just those undergoing IVF.

By the time you have finished reading this book, I hope I have inspired you, and given you the confidence to take control of your health and implement positive changes in the hope that one day you may be blessed with your own bundle of joy.

Section 1

Infertility & IVF

This section looks at the causes of infertility in women and men, and some of the fertility tests you may both have to undertake. It also provides you with a high-level overview of the IVF process and what happens at each stage of the cycle.

Finally, it looks at how naturopathic therapies can prepare and support you and your partner on your IVF journey.

Notes

CAUSES OF INFERTILITY

Making a baby sounds relatively simple – a couple of ingredients from both partners, the correct 'cooking time' and you should have a bouncing bundle of joy about 40 weeks later. For many couples, this dream seems unachievable and can lead to feelings of inadequacy, bitter disappointment and heartbreak.

Infertility is defined as the failure to conceive after one year of regular unprotected sex. As many as one in seven couples may have difficulty conceiving. In the UK, that is around 3.5 million people.

Fortunately, Assisted Reproductive Technologies (ART) such as IVF can help. The good news is there are effective naturopathic treatment methods to complement this intensive process that can maximise your chances of success.

The villains of infertility

There are many causes of infertility in men and women, ranging from hormonal disturbances, autoimmune diseases, congenital abnormalities to infection, oxidative stress and, sadly, unexplained reasons. In both sexes, there are common drivers underlying these factors. In many cases, it comes back to the same old villains that naturopaths see every day: obesity, stress, a toxic lifestyle and poor diet, mixed with the patient's unique genetic tendencies.

Unexplained infertility occurs in approximately five to ten per cent of couples trying to conceive. They may have problems with egg quality, tubal function or sperm function that are difficult to diagnose and treat.

In some cases, the likelihood of unexplained infertility being a true diagnosis reflects poor investigation to accurately determine the cause. These couples are often directed to the easiest solution - IVF – without always assessing what may actually be causing the problem.

This is why a holistic approach to fertility is beneficial as often naturopaths can help identify more subtle causes of infertility which have previously been diagnosed as unexplained.

Infertility causes in women and men

Infertility is not just a female issue. In approximately 40 per cent of infertile couples, the problem is a male factor. In about 40 per cent it is a female factor, in 10 per cent it is a joint problem and in the remaining 10 per cent the cause is unknown.

Some causes of female infertility

Ovulation disorders account for up to 40 per cent of female infertility. This is due to:

- Ageing
- Diminished ovarian reserve (low AMH)
- Hypothalamic amenorrhoea
- Hyperprolactinemia
- Thyroid disease
- Adrenal disease
- Polycystic Ovarian Syndrome (PCOS)
- Premature ovarian failure.

Uterine (womb) and fallopian tube problems account for up to 30 per cent of female infertility issues. This is due to:

- Obstruction due to pelvic inflammatory disease or tubal surgery
- Previous ectopic pregnancy
- Pelvic inflammatory disorder
- Infection
- Fibroids
- Endometriosis (accounting for up to 15 per cent of causes) and sometimes subsequent uterine adhesions resulting in Asherman's syndrome
- Polyps on the endometrial lining

- Congenital structural issues with the uterus.

Other issues that account for up to 10 per cent of female infertility include:

- Poor cervical mucous quantity and/or quality (may be due to smoking, infection)
- Mucous hostility to sperm
- Certain medications.

A large amount of women's issues are related to issues with oestrogen metabolism, an area where naturopathic treatment can be very successful.

Some causes of male infertility

The primary issues below account for up to 30 to 40 per cent of male infertility:

- Hormone imbalance (mainly issues with testosterone, but also prolactin and other hormones)
- Congenital or developmental testicular disorder (e.g. Klinefelter syndrome)
- Cryptorchidism (undescended testes)
- Certain medications.

Altered sperm transport account for up to 10 to 20 per cent of male infertility. This is due to:

- Structural abnormalities
- Obstruction
- Infections
- Injury e.g. spinal cord injury
- Surgery (including vasectomy or vasectomy reversal).

Immune issues such as infection, inflammation, sperm antibodies and autoimmune disease can contribute to male infertility. Chromosome defects can also contribute to sperm defects.

Up to 40 to 50 per cent of male infertility causes are unknown and are perhaps related to:

- Issues with sperm quality, sometimes the absence of sperm
- Ageing
- Obesity
- Radiation exposure
- Genito-urinary infection
- Excessive heat
- Heavy metal toxicity
- Poor nutritional status
- Cigarette smoking
- Pesticide exposure
- High intake of cottonseed oil
- Environmental oestrogen exposure.

Other causes may include:

- Mumps
- Testicular trauma
- Varicocele
- Tumour.

More information on male infertility can be found in the *The Diet Guide for Men.*

INVESTIGATIONS AND ASSESSMENTS

If you are reading this book, you and your partner have no doubt had countless investigations and blood tests (unless you are using donor egg or sperm).

For women

You may have been through the mill already and had a laparoscopy, hysteroscopy, salpingoscopy and/or ultrasound scan alongside hormone blood tests.

Your doctor/reproductive specialist should have also already conducted tests for:

- Rubella antibodies
- Hepatitis B surface antigen
- HIV antibody/antigen
- Hepatitis C antibody
- Chlamydia
- Toxoplasmosis, CMV, EBV
- Pap smear test
- Cervical swab
- Urine analysis.

They may also request:

- Miscarriage panel if appropriate (such as Karyotype 46XX, thrombophilia)
- Sperm antibodies (serum).
- Here is a checklist to make sure you have also had these tests conducted:
- Day 1-5 ovarian reserve test: includes Follicle Stimulating Hormone (FSH), luteinising hormone (LH), oestradiol and prolactin. Usually more than one test is performed as levels tend to fluctuate, particularly those of FSH and oestradiol.
- Day 3 fertility potential test: includes Anti-Mullerian and Inhibin B hormone tests

- Testosterone (free and bound)
- Sex Hormone Binding Globulin (SHBG)
- Thyroid function test: thyroid stimulating hormone (TSH), thyroxine (T4), triiodothyronine (T3), Reverse T3 and thyroid antibodies
- Day 21 Progesterone
- Menstrual blood analysis to detect bacteria such as Chlamydia or other infectious microorganisms. Such detection in menstrual blood allows the diagnosis of both active and hidden/dormant states of Chlamydial infections, which is difficult to detect by conventional methods of testing.

In addition, your doctor or naturopath may request:

- Full blood count (FBC) and blood type test
- Folate and vitamin B12 blood test
- MTHFR genetic test (especially if there is a history of miscarriage)
- Vitamin D blood test
- Liver function test (LFT)
- Electrolyte blood test
- Iron studies
- Fasting glucose test if indicated
- Coeliac screen/gluten antibody test.
- Sometimes, if relevant, your naturopath may also request:
- Salivary hormone screen to include E1, E2, E3, progesterone and testosterone, DHEA, cortisol and melatonin
- 2 and 16 urinary oestrogen metabolism tests
- Nutrient and toxic screening
- Environmental screening (heavy metals toxicity, pesticides, other chemicals).

For men

Your partner's doctor usually conducts a semen analysis, blood test, urine analysis and sexually transmitted infection (STI) screen. A naturopath may also request your partner be tested for heavy metals, environmental toxins and saliva hormone analysis. Refer to *The Diet Guide for Men* for more details.

Notes

THE INS AND OUTS OF IVF

Depending on the underlying cause(s) of infertility, your doctor may offer one of the following options to help you conceive:

- Surgery (for example, when endometriosis is suspected)
- Hormonal treatment
- Ovulation induction with Clomiphene Citrate (Clomid)
- Assisted Reproductive Technologies (ART) treatment, one of which is IVF.

Looked at simply, these procedures can firstly increase the number of eggs released in any one cycle (in IVF it can be several eggs). These techniques can also shorten the distance between your eggs and your partner's sperm, optimising fertilisation opportunities.

Fertilisation can take place inside or outside the body, depending on which procedure is used:

- IUI (Intra-uterine Insemination): the sperm is put in the uterus (womb) so fertilisation takes place inside the body.
- GIFT (Gamete Intra Fallopian Transfer): the sperm and egg are mixed together outside the body but fertilisation takes place inside the body.
- IVF: the sperm and egg are mixed together and fertilised outside the body.
- ICSI (Intracytoplasmic Sperm Injection): the sperm is put inside the egg outside the body.

I have chosen to focus on the most common ART procedure - IVF. For more detailed information on IVF and other ART procedures, please contact your fertility clinic.

When IVF begins

Generally, after one year of trying to conceive without success, women (and ideally their male partner) will be offered further medical investigations by their doctor. However, women with known factors that put them at high risk of infertility (such as certain cancer treatments) will be referred to a fertility clinic straightaway. Otherwise, IVF is only offered to women in many countries including the UK after two years or more of trying to conceive.

The IVF procedure

IVF is a technique for fertilising your eggs with your partner's sperm (or donor sperm) outside your body, hence the use of the phrase 'test tube babies'. The fertilised egg is then implanted into your uterus.

What happens?

To prepare your body for IVF, you may be given GnRH (Gonadotrophin Releasing Hormone) analogues, either as a nasal spray or daily injection, to suppress your natural monthly cycle (unless you have hypothalamic amenorrhoea and other conditions that stop a menstrual cycle). This is called down-regulation and stops your hormones interfering with the IVF treatment.

You will then be injected with another fertility drug, FSH (follicle stimulating hormone) or HMG (Human Menopausal Gonadotrophin), to stimulate several follicles to develop. The FSH is a daily injection that you give yourself to boost the number of eggs in the ovaries, so more eggs can be retrieved and fertilised, giving doctors a greater choice of embryos.

You are then monitored with blood tests to check oestrogen levels, and ultrasounds to determine the number of follicles developing and growing. Once there are enough follicles of the correct size, you are injected with HCG (an ovulation trigger injection) which primes the eggs (helps them mature) before they are collected.

Around 34 to 48 hours after the HCG injection the egg retrieval takes place. The eggs are collected through the vagina, using an aspiration needle guided by ultrasound. You may be sedated for this procedure or have a general anaesthetic.

Your partner provides a fresh semen sample, which is washed and centrifuged so that the weaker sperm are filtered out, and up to

100,000 sperm are mixed with each egg. An embryologist (IVF scientist) fertilises the eggs with your partner's or donor sperm. The eggs that are fertilised, and start to divide well, will be transferred back inside the uterus. This takes place two to five days later (depending on quantity and quality). The embryo(s) are transferred into the uterus via the cervix, using a soft catheter.

The country you live in will determine how many embryos can be implanted. In the UK, clinics can transfer a maximum of two embryos in women under the age of 40 years and three embryos in women of 40 years and above. In Australia, single embryo transfer is usually recommended unless you are over 40 years old, where a maximum of two embryos are transferred. European countries are similar. For the US, the guidelines state that doctors can consider transferring up to four or five embryos in women 40 and older, although this is less common.

To increase the chances of implantation, you will be given the hormone progesterone either as pessaries, gel or injection to prepare for and support implantation and to reduce uterine irritability. A special series of three HCG injections are often administered over the first few days after egg retrieval. Sometimes oral oestrogen can be added to progesterone during the luteal phase in agonist cycles to further assist pregnancy and implantation rates. Then it is a waiting game until the pregnancy test day!

Assisted hatching

If there have been a number of failed attempts at IVF, a technique called assisted hatching may be used, whereby a needle or chemical is used to make a tiny hole in the casing of the embryo to help it hatch and attach itself to the uterine lining.

Frozen embryos

Extra embryos resulting from the IVF treatment can be frozen if their quality is good. They are stored in liquid nitrogen and, to prevent what is called 'cooling injury' as the embryos are thawed out, cryoprotectant chemicals are used. There are moral and ethical issues that must be considered when deciding whether to freeze embryos, because it is not eggs that are being frozen but a potential baby.

Be patient

IVF is a fairly lengthy process. It can be very stressful, and the success rates are not always what you think they might be.

Measure of success

The most important outcome measure of any IVF treatment is the birth of a healthy baby to a healthy mother. Such outcomes are referred to as live birth or delivery rates.

The statistics

Regardless of the country, statistics will vary from clinic to clinic. Many factors contribute to the success of an IVF procedure. Some factors are related to the training and experience of the IVF clinic and laboratory professionals and the quality of services they provide. Other factors are related to the patients themselves, such as their age and the cause of their infertility. Some clinics may be more willing than others to accept patients with low chances of success or may specialise in various ART treatments that attract particular types of patients.

The US Center for Disease Control and Prevention estimates that 1.5 per cent of babies born in the US are conceived using ART, of which the most common procedure is IVF. About 36 per cent of IVF cycles result in pregnancy, and 29 per cent of cycles result in a baby.[1]

[1] uk.businessinsider.com/ivf-success-rates-2015

A live birth rate of about 30 per cent for IVF cycles is fairly respectable. A healthy, fertile 30-year-old woman has about a 20 per cent chance of getting pregnant without assistance every month that she tries. That decreases to 5 per cent each month for women aged 40.

To put that IVF success data in a slightly different frame, however, most IVF cycles do not result in pregnancy. The flipside of a 36 per cent pregnancy rate is that 64 per cent of IVF cycles don't result in pregnancy.

A woman undergoing IVF may have a better chance of getting pregnant than she would without the procedure, but it's nowhere near a sure thing.

Age Matters

A woman's age is the most important factor influencing the success of IVF when she uses her own eggs. Around 40 per cent of IVF cycles result in babies for women aged 32 and younger. Not even 10 years later, for women aged 40, that success rate is cut in half to less than 20 per cent.

While looking at averages for IVF success rates, remember these statistics can't possibly predict what will happen for each individual patient. There are many different causes of infertility, and IVF does not address the direct problem for every cause. Only your doctor can say what chance IVF has of success for you.

Don't let these statistics discourage you. By taking control of your health and wellbeing before and during your IVF treatment, you may help improve your chances of conceiving and having a healthy pregnancy.

When IVF doesn't work

In some instances, sadly, IVF may not be successful due to factors such as:

- Ovarian problems: poor ovarian response, few follicles, reduced quality of eggs
- Sperm factors: poor sperm health (quality, count, motility, morphology, although with ICSI this factor is less relevant)
- Uterine factors: thin uterine lining, poor receptivity of the endometrial lining (thus low implantation rate)
- Embryonic factors: poor embryo quality (embryos that do not divide sufficiently or disintegrate early), embryo not viable leading to miscarriage.

There are no guarantees that IVF will work, with or without complementary holistic support. But have hope that maybe one day, you will be blessed with a healthy pregnancy and a healthy baby.

HOLISTIC IVF NATUROPATHIC SUPPORT

Naturopathy is a system of healthcare that emphasises optimal wellness, disease prevention, patient education and the use of natural medicine to support the body's inherent healing process.

Naturopathic philosophy focuses on optimising and aiming to restore your body to its natural state or, from a Traditional Chinese Medicine (TCM) view, strengthening the 'chi' or 'vital force' (the body's innate ability to heal itself).

Naturopaths use a holistic approach to establish the root cause of your problem. Usually a naturopath will devise a specific treatment plan including diet and lifestyle advice to help you reach optimal health. In addition, nutritional medicine, mineral therapy, herbal and homoeopathic medicines and flower essences may be prescribed. Your naturopath may also provide some counselling and visualisation techniques.

Naturopaths place a lot of emphasis on preconception care including detoxification and nutrition repletion, treating both the female and male (if using your partner's sperm). But it isn't just about supporting the reproductive system; a naturopath also supports the various systems (e.g. nervous system, digestive system, adrenal glands) that work to address your fertility.

When IVF is the only option

IVF provides treatment for patients that no other treatment can offer. It is especially relevant for couples who have physical or genetic impediments that prevent natural conception. There are some couples/people that naturopaths just can't help, which is why we're lucky to have IVF technology available.

When a patient would like to combine holistic naturopathic support with IVF, the relationship must be one of mutual respect and collaboration.

The following table demonstrates how naturopathy and TCM including acupuncture can benefit and support the IVF process.

Combined approach to treatment

Timeline	IVF	Naturopathy	TCM
Pre-conception	Investigations, medications	Investigations, preconceptual treatment with nutritional supplementation, herbal medicine, lifestyle, diet	Investigations, preconceptual treatment with acupuncture, herbal medicine, lifestyle, diet
Ovarian stimulation	Clomiphene citrate (Clomid)/FSH Ovarian drilling	Nutritional supplementation, herbal medicine, lifestyle, diet	Acupuncture, herbal medicine, lifestyle, diet
Long cycle	Contraceptive pill	Nutritional supplementation, herbal medicine, lifestyle, diet	Acupuncture, herbal medicine, lifestyle, diet
Stimulation	FSH injections	Nutritional supplementation, diet, lifestyle, limited herbal medicine use	Acupuncture, diet, lifestyle
LH surge prevention	GnRH analogues, GnRH agonists, GnRH antagonists	Nutritional supplementation, diet, lifestyle	Acupuncture, diet, lifestyle
Triggering Ovulation	Human Chorionic Gonadotrophin (HCG) injections		Acupuncture
Egg collection	Additional treatment if required	Nutritional supplementation, diet, lifestyle	Acupuncture
Sperm collection	Additional treatment if required	Treatment of male pre-conceptually as required	Treatment of male pre-conceptually as required

Embryo culture	Patience and support	Diet, lifestyle, limited herbal medicine depending on recommendations	Acupuncture, diet, lifestyle, limited herbal medicine depending on recommendations
Transferring embryos	May involve blood thinners, hormone modulators, corticosteroids	Diet, lifestyle, limited herbal medicine depending on recommendations	Acupuncture, diet, lifestyle, limited herbal medicine depending on recommendations
Endometrial support	HCG (Pregnyl shots), progesterone	Nutritional supplementation, diet, lifestyle, herbal medicine depending on recommendations	Acupuncture, diet, lifestyle, herbal medicine depending on recommendations
Pregnancy test	Cheer or start again	Cheer, more patient management and/or start again	Cheer, more patient management and/or start again

Table adapted from Lyttleton, J.,2004, Treatment of Infertility with Chinese Medicine, Churchill Livingstone and Fertility Masterclass Seminar by L Hechtman, Sydney 2012

Integrative treatment

The following table also reflects the holistic combination of IVF with naturopathy and TCM treatment support.

Requirement	IVF	Naturopathy	TCM
Preconception support		✓	✓
Improve egg and sperm quality		✓	✓
Improve fertilisation potential	✓	✓	✓
Optimise embryo quality	✓	✓	✓
Optimise endometrial lining for implantation	✓	✓	✓
Viable pregnancy with good birth rates	✓	✓	✓
Consider miscarriage factors	✓	✓	✓

Table adapted from Lyttleton, J.,2004, Treatment of Infertility with Chinese Medicine, Churchill Livingstone and Fertility Masterclass Seminar by L Hechtman, Sydney 2012

Section 2

Three-Step IVF Pre-conception Preparation Plan

Preconception (also referred to as pre-fertilisation) can be seen as the ultimate form of preventative medicine.

The naturopathic aim of preconception healthcare is simply to optimise the general and reproductive health of both partners to ensure the health of the egg and sperm and a nurturing environment for your developing baby.

This aim is to not just improve you and your partner's health, but to also positively influence your baby's health and their babies – not one, but two subsequent generations.

Ploughing the field

You are about to embark on one of the most important journeys of your life - the creation of a new, unique and very special little person. This is a very exciting and sometimes, an overwhelming time. You *can* have a very positive effect on your fertility and IVF success, the course of your pregnancy, the birth and the health of your baby by making wise and informative lifestyle and dietary choices. This is very important for both parents, particularly during the preconception phase.

A three-month preconception preparation plan

There is a critical four-month window for an ideal preconception diet and lifestyle programme to be implemented. Why? Egg development takes 100 days and sperm 80 days. The health of the egg and sperm reflect the health of the environment in which they grow. The instant the egg and sperm combine, an irreversible genetic code is formed for the future development of your baby.

Early nutrition determines adult disease

Compelling evidence reveals the programming of much of our future health begins in the months before birth. A key trigger in this process is the nutritional supply reaching the developing baby (foetus).

Foetal programming begins in the first to second week of embryo development.

Since we have the environmental capacity to affect gene outcomes (the study of epigenetics), the mother's nutrition is vital.

Better health in-utero, better health overall!

A general IVF cycle is around six weeks from the beginning of medications and ultrasounds to the embryo(s) being transferred, so if time permits, it makes sense to plan accordingly.

You (and your partner if you are not using donor sperm) should plan and prepare for your IVF procedure at least three months before it is due to take place. The cycle of the egg (ovum) is 90 days. This is the period of time during the egg's journey when what you eat, drink and breathe, your stress levels, and the health of your blood flow will all have an effect on the health of the egg three months down the track.

Since the follicles contain the fluid filled with nutrients that help support the egg development, it makes sense to address your health leading up to the IVF cycle to maximise your chance of success.

Since the development and maturation of sperm takes approximately 80 days, it makes sense for your partner to also embark on a preconception preparation plan. Please refer to *The Diet Guide for Men* for more information.

A three-step preconception preparation plan

1. Preconception detox and cleanse

Gentle detoxification and cleansing are an important part of preparing for conception and pregnancy. I recommend a supervised detoxification programme as a first step for prospective parents: removing any pathogenic bacteria and toxins, then replenishing the gut with beneficial bacteria, like probiotics, while simultaneously supporting liver function and elimination. By taking such steps you are giving your body the best chance to be in optimal health. This in turn can support hormonal health and encourage a healthy uterine environment.

2. Preconception diet plan

The second part of the preparation plan focuses on supporting egg health, eating specific, nutritious food and incorporating nutritional medicine to prepare your body for conception and pregnancy.

A vast amount of nutritional research states that a woman in an optimal state of health will increase her odds of conception and a healthier pregnancy.

3. Preconception lifestyle and stress support

The final part of the preparation plan provides lifestyle strategies such as exercise, weight loss advice and specific therapies to help you manage the stress that may be experienced once you begin IVF medications and procedures.

PRECONCEPTION DETOX AND CLEANSE

Getting rid of toxins in the body, which often come from cigarettes, alcohol, environmental oestrogens, pesticides, food preservatives, heavy metals, medications and synthetic hormones can affect both male and female infertility.

The problem is such suspect toxins seem to be everywhere – in the food we eat, the air we breathe, and the things we use at work and at home. We can avoid many of them and minimise our exposure to others. But we obviously cannot completely eliminate them, short of finding a non-polluted island where we can live and eat organically forever more.

However, reducing your exposure is only part of the plan. There are plenty of ways to protect yourself against the unavoidable exposure to toxins and to ensure they are effectively eliminated from your system.

It therefore makes sense to do a gentle detox to prepare for IVF and encourage healthy hormone balance and optimal health in preparation for pregnancy.

Managing environmental toxins

Think about your environment. Could your occupation or your partner's be affecting fertility (e.g. farming with pesticides, hairdressing with dyes and hairspray, or painting)? And can you do anything to reduce the problem?

In your home, can you limit the amount of chemicals used? For example, can you avoid using pesticides in the garden and pest sprays in the house? If you are decorating the house, finish the work before you begin a preconception plan.

Chemicals are everywhere, creating havoc with our hormones, namely oestrogen. Here are some of the toxins you may be faced with.

Endogenous toxins

The body creates endogenous toxins during the metabolism process. These toxins are known as free radicals. When free radical production exceeds antioxidant intake, cellular damage occurs.

Exogenous toxins

These are the poisonous by-products that the body ingests but cannot neutralise. They include alcohol, tobacco, caffeine, recreational drugs, over-the-counter medicines, hair bleach, and non-organic skin care.

Environmental toxins

The most damaging environmental toxins include radiation, pesticides, fungicides, herbicides, petrochemicals, exhaust fumes, chlorine, heavy metals (e.g. mercury), and environmental oestrogens (from dairy and non-organic farming). These toxins poison the cells and tissues directly.

Radiation

We can be exposed to ionising radiation so easily via x-rays and flying. Research has shown that sperm morphology and increased miscarriage rates can be affected by a single lower body x-ray, for up to three years after the event! The other source of ionising radiation is the cosmic radiation we are exposed to at high altitudes, for example when flying on commercial flights, with one four-hour flight at 32,000 feet being equivalent of one chest x-ray.

Mobile phones

Mobile phones carried close to the lower body (e.g. in trouser pockets) can affect the health of the ovaries in women and testes in men. Try not to carry your mobile phone in your back pocket! What's more, when left on at night in the bedroom, they can prevent delta wave deep (restorative) sleep.

Microwave radiation

Microwave ovens emit an extremely large electromagnetic field and destroy proteins and the enzymes required to absorb vitamins and minerals. Stand in the next room if you have to use one.

In the bedroom

Electromagnetic pollution is everywhere. Just look at the bedroom - people sleep with their mobile phone next to their heads on their bedside table, along with clock radios, televisions and tablets left to charge overnight. The use of electric blankets and water beds have even been linked male fertility problems and increased miscarriage rates.

Protect yourself from radiation

The best place to protect is the bedroom, where we spend about a third of our lives, and when, during sleep, cells are at their most vulnerable. Sleep free of active appliances, turn off power points, and get your mobile phone out of the bedroom!

Increase eating foods that protect the body from radiation, such as superfoods including acai, kelp and seaweed (great sources of iodine), chlorella, spirulina, blue-green algae, miso, bee pollen, royal jelly, hemp and goji berries. Other beneficial foods include leafy green vegetables, garlic, onion, asparagus, pineapple, watermelon, turmeric and high pectin foods (apple, guava, plums and citrus fruits).

Caution: foods coming from radiation disaster areas are contaminated. Beware of business interests covering this up - know your food sources.

Your naturopath may also prescribe zeolites, antioxidants, multi-mineral supplements, and herbs such as Astragalus, Ginseng, Echinacea and Rhodiola.

Environmental chemicals

Environmental exposure to the many chemicals listed below can adversely affect your hormone balance, thyroid health and fertility. Unfortunately, much of the medical profession and the general public remain largely unaware of the effects these dangerous chemicals are exerting on our lives and those of animals.

Chemicals including parabens found in deodorants, dioxins present in tampons, chlorine bleaches, petrol combustion by-products, and pesticides such as dieldrin, atrazine and methylchlor are all of major concern to the reproductive health of women.

Phthalates - present in seatbelts, hose pipes, plastic dental fillings, lubricants, moisturisers, hairsprays, insect repellents, solvents, coatings on time-released medicines, children's toys, food packaging, soap, shampoo and detergents. They can enter the body via food and water, through the skin and inhaled from polluted air. DEHP (di-ethyl hexyl phthalate), one of the most abundantly used phthalates, has been measured in blood and shown to decrease LH, increase FSH and delay ovulation.

Bisphenol A (BPA) – plasticisers present in flexible plastics e.g. PVC and polycarbonate plastics, cellophane, cling wrap/cling film, some dental materials, plastic bags, polystyrene cups, takeaway containers and linings in food cans. Increased temperatures and storage can cause BPA to leach into our food, enter our bodies and bind to oestrogen receptors. It has also been detected in human follicular fluid (bathes the egg as it grows and develops). Exposure to BPA is associated with recurrent miscarriages and the presence of antinuclear antibodies. Studies have reported women undergoing IVF have up to 95 per cent quantifiable levels of BPA. High BPA levels in women decrease the chance of IVF being successful.

Thankfully it is now possible to buy storage and beverage containers that are BPA-free.

Organochloride Compounds (OCCs) – and many other pesticides including insecticides, fungicides and herbicides have been linked to decreased ovulation, impaired implantation, altered uterine function, and reduced semen quality in men. Exposure during fertilisation can also affect the development of the embryo.[2] Exposure is primarily from the consumption of contaminated animal products, water and breast milk.

Organic solvents - people working in the clothing, textiles, paint and plastic industries, and healthcare professionals and laboratory workers are exposed to organic solvents. These may impair fertility and increase the risk of miscarriage and major malformations.

Heavy metals – such as lead, mercury, cadmium, arsenic and nickel are present in cigarette smoke, paints, plastics, batteries, water pipes, dental fillings, fluorescent lights, large fish, cosmetics and treated pine. Lead crosses the placenta easily and affects the hormonal environment needed to maintain pregnancy. An even low level of lead exposure is associated with increased risk of miscarriage and still birth. Mercury exposure has been identified in dental assistants preparing amalgams and is also linked to miscarriage and reduced fertility.

Pharmaceutical drugs – such as Cyclophosphamide have been linked to premature ovarian failure. Non-Steroidal Anti Inflammatories (NSAIDS) and COX-2 inhibitors may interfere with ovulation and miscarriage. A recent study has proven that NSAIDs also dramatically reduce ovulation with consistent use.[3]

[2] Tiemann U. Reprod Toxic 2008; 25:316-326
[3] Medscape 15 June 2015

Protect yourself from environmental toxicity

Enhancing liver detoxification pathways and optimising antioxidant status is critical to reduce the toxic burden of many chemicals, as is eating a wholefood, antioxidant-rich diet.

Your naturopath may also recommend:

- Amino acids such as glutamine, glycine, taurine, cysteine, methionine and choline, and chelaters such as humic acid, vitamin C and glutathione
- Coriander – protects against mercury toxicity
- Herbs such as garlic, milk thistle, rosemary, schizandra and turmeric to support liver detoxification by improving overall liver health
- Herbal teas such as dandelion and nettle to aid both detoxification and to encourage regular bowel movements
- More traditional naturopathic remedies such as aloe vera and liquid chlorophyll (refer to my detox drink below)
- Oil pulling

Many of these nutrients and herbs can be found combined in specific detox formulas.

Body Care

Dry skin brushing can boost circulation and improve lymphatic drainage.

Epsom salt baths are a traditional remedy for increasing circulation and drawing out toxins.

Skincare

Do you read the labels of your skincare and haircare products? Every year, new toxic chemicals are developed and incorporated into our moisturisers, makeup and hair dyes. Sixty per cent of what we coat our skin with ends up in our bloodstream. On average, women are exposed to over 500 different chemicals from their skin and haircare before leaving the house!

Avoid ingredients that sound unnatural. Some common chemicals to avoid include parabens (Butylparaben, Ethylparaben, Isobutylparaben and Isopropylparaben), phthalates (Di-butyl-phthalate, Di-ethylhexyl-phthalate), petroleum by-products (Petrolatum, Paraffin, Dipropylene, Glycol, Butylene), sodium laurel/laureth sulphate, Diethanolamine (DEA), Triethanolamine (TEA), and Formaldehyde (Diazolindyl, Imidazolindyl urea).

Instead, focus on organic skincare products or get creative and make your own. The simplest, most natural body moisturiser? Coconut oil with a splash of your favourite essential oil.

Preconception detox tips

Ideally a preconception detox is based on your monthly cycle and generally lasts from 25 to 30 days (although your naturopath may suggest a three-month detox depending on your circumstances). Doing a detox at least three months before IVF treatment is recommended. However, if time does not permit this, try the following 'express detox' alongside my detox cocktail and 'oil pulling'.

The 10 golden rules for an 'express detox'

1. Do not eat between 6 p.m. and 7 a.m.
2. Avoid ALL refined sugar, such as cakes, biscuits and sweets.
3. Avoid wheat and dairy.
4. Drink plenty of filtered water.
5. Avoid alcohol.
6. Eat regular servings of light protein foods balanced with high-fibre vegetables.
7. Start the day with warm water and lemon juice.
8. Take supplements such as probiotics, B vitamins, selenium, milk thistle and turmeric (for more details, refer to Section 5, Supplements).
9. Exercise daily.
10. Sleep eight hours per night.

Try my detox cocktail

This is a great detox cocktail – drink every morning for six weeks.

In a large glass of water, add:

- 1 dessertspoon liquid chlorophyll
- 1–2 dessertspoons aloe vera juice
- 1 dessertspoon psyllium husks.

Stir and drink immediately, followed by another glass of water.

Liquid chlorophyll acts as an internal deodoriser and a 'prebiotic' to help support beneficial gut bacteria. Aloe vera is a soothing, healing plant that helps eliminate toxins, especially if you are prone to constipation. Psyllium husks provide dietary fibre and help to bind and excrete toxins. Just think of these husks as an 'intestinal' broom.

Detox with oil pulling

The ancient Ayurvedic practice of oil pulling – swishing a tablespoon of coconut oil around your mouth each day - is enjoying a resurgence, and for good reason. It has been linked to better weight control and digestion, improvements in immunity and metabolism, clarity of mind, fewer headaches and allergies, hormone balancing and even minimising fine lines and wrinkles. Oil pulling is like the function of your car's motor oil, where the oil absorbs debris in the engine which is then removed when the oil is changed.

A window to your body

According to Ayurvedic medical theory, oral health not only affects teeth and gums but also a person's entire body and vigour: meridians (energy pathways) on the tongue are linked to every organ in the body, and when you swish oil around the tongue you soothe and stimulate these organs. Oil pulling as we know it today was introduced in a scientific paper in 1992 by Dr F. Karach, who claimed it had cured him of a chronic blood disease that he had suffered from for 15 years. His findings stirred up worldwide interest in the technique.

Traditionally, sesame or sunflower oil was used, but coconut oil is the modern oil of choice because of the naturally occurring anti-microbial, anti-bacterial and anti-fungal lauric acid.

The mouth is home to billions of micro-organisms, most of them bacteria. Some have the potential to be pathogenic (disease causing), and an unhealthy mouth can become a gateway to the bloodstream for them. These organisms can cause systemic and localised infections, chronic inflammation, and autoimmune responses that can lead to many health problems.

Sucking and swishing coconut oil around the mouth is supposed to pull pathogens and toxins out from around the gums and teeth. When you spit out the oil, the pathogens and toxins leave your body. This lessens the load on your immune system, making it easier for the body to heal itself.

DIY oil pulling

1. Immediately upon rising, and on an empty stomach, put a tablespoon of coconut oil in your mouth and let it melt.

2. Swish the oil around your mouth, sucking it through your teeth for 20 minutes.

3. Spit the oil out into a rubbish bin. It should be white.

4. Rinse mouth with warm salt water, and brush teeth thoroughly.

Note: Never swallow the oil because it may be loaded with toxins.

Notes

PRECONCEPTION DIET PLAN

It takes roughly 80 days for sperm to mature and up to four months before an egg is ovulated and presented for possible fertilisation. These two facts make it easy to see that preconceptual nutrition planning is vital to the health of your future bundle of joy.

> Some great mantras by Michael Pollan, author of *In Defence of Food: An Eater's Manifesto*:
>
> *"Eat food. Not too much. Mostly plants."*
>
> *"Don't eat anything your great-grandmother wouldn't recognise as food."*
>
> *"Don't eat anything incapable of rotting."*

Recommended preconception diet guidelines

Here are my seven preconception diet guidelines.

Eat organic

Herbicides, pesticides and fungicides are rife in our non-organic food chain. Whenever possible, focus on organic produce. Ideally, eat seasonally and locally produced foods as much as possible. If sourcing organic products is difficult, consider signing up for a weekly delivery of organic vegetables and fruits, or seek out local farmers' markets.

If cost is an issue, wash non-organic fruit and vegetables thoroughly with a vegetable wash, Citricidal (grapefruit seed extract) or vinegar to remove nasty compounds from the skin. Washing cannot alter the amount of pesticides absorbed into the fruit and vegetables, but peeling can lower the pesticide residues by about three-quarters.

The 'clean fifteen' foods below have been found to contain the least amount of pesticides by the US-based Environmental Working Group, while the 'dirty dozen' contain high levels of pesticides.

Clean Fifteen	Dirty Dozen
Onions	Apples
Sweet corn	Celery
Pineapple	Strawberries
Avocado	Peaches
Asparagus	Spinach
Snow peas (mange tout)	Nectarines
Mangoes	Grapes
Eggplant (aubergine)	Capsicum (bell peppers)
Rockmelon (cantaloupe)	Potatoes
Kiwi	Blueberries
Cabbage	Lettuce
Watermelon	Kale
Sweet potato (kumura)	
Grapefruit	
Mushrooms	

Clean fifteen/dirty dozen (www.ewg.org)

Increase your antioxidant intake

Antioxidants are our internal defence mechanism against toxins and cellular damage. 'Eat a rainbow' as the saying goes, adding to your diet nuts, seeds, berries and an array of different-coloured produce to ensure you have the widest possible range of nutrients. You may like to add antioxidant-rich superfoods and vegetable juices for an extra boost.

Consume alkaline foods to maintain a healthy pH

Most of our body fluids like blood, urine, saliva, cervical secretions and semen have an alkaline pH. Our body does its best to maintain a healthy pH, but if we constantly eat acid-forming foods, your body will be more prone to inflammation, calcium loss from the bones and kidney stress. Acid foods include sugar, red meat, excess refined grains, tea, coffee, alcohol and soft drinks. Alkalising foods include fruit and vegetables, especially leafy greens. Think 'green smoothies' and superfoods! One of the most alkaline fruits is lemon so starting the day with a slice of lemon in hot water is a great way to kickstart your body, especially your liver!

Support gut bacteria (microbiome)

Looking after your gut health is essential for maintaining optimal health. We carry up to three kilograms of gut bacteria in our digestive system (gut). Beneficial bacteria usually live harmoniously among potentially harmful bacteria such as E-coli, thankfully outweighing the harmful bacteria. But it is more than just bacteria that colonises in our gut; candida, yeasts, fungi and even parasites can be found in our digestive system. For this reason, this community of gut organisms is more commonly referred to as the gut 'microbiota'.

Scientifically speaking, the gut microbiome, the term used to describe the complex ecosystem within your digestive system, is inextricably linked to your overall wellbeing. An altered gut microbiome can trigger all types of problems, from food cravings to depression, and even an increased risk of developing an autoimmune disorder.

The good guys (good microbiota organisms) help maintain healthy digestion (including regular bowel movements), manufacture K and B vitamins and help to metabolise oestrogen. Good bacteria are critical for the health of our immune system and play an important role in reducing inflammation.

Beneficial foods to encourage the growth of good bacteria and maintain a healthy microbiota balance include 'prebiotics', which consist of herbs such as aloe vera and slippery elm; fibre-rich fruit and vegetables (including onion, garlic, leek, broccoli and cauliflower stalks); seeds; nuts; chicory; and fermented foods such as yoghurt, kefir, sauerkraut, miso and kimchi (a Korean fermented vegetable dish).

Minimise unnecessary toxins from food in your diet

It may be hard to avoid exhaust fumes, atmospheric carbon dioxide and petrochemicals, but you can control what you eat, including meat and dairy.

An area of much controversy is the high concentration of hormones and antibiotics in dairy and meat products. Cattle are exposed to frequent rounds of antibiotics to keep them disease-free, fast-growing and in the case of cows, yielding high quantities of milk. At least two-thirds of non-organic milk is extracted from pregnant cows. This contributes to considerably higher levels or oestrogen and antibiotics in milk, which may lead to hormonal and immunological changes when consumed in significant quantities.

Our bodies struggle to detoxify these hormones and antibiotics. Whenever possible, avoid non-organic dairy, meat and fish and experiment with nourishing non-dairy milks, such as almond, hemp and rice milk. If you can't resist the occasional steak, make sure it is grass-fed and organic.

Avoid GM foods

Genetically modified (GM) foods should be avoided at all costs. Genetic modification means that genes from another species can be introduced into a particular plant, usually to make it more resistant to pests, viruses, weedkillers or other hazards – in other words, tampering with nature. For instance, you can buy tomatoes which contain a fish gene to boost its resistance to frost. The gene is from a flounder because they survive well in cold water. This same flounder gene has also been introduced into some farmed salmon to speed up their growth rate. Another example of a popular GM food is soy. Up to 60 per cent of processed foods contain soy, including bread, biscuits and baby food.

There are worries that GM foods will make various diseases resistant to life-saving antibiotics. This is another reason to buy organic and to read your labels carefully.

Cook and store your food carefully

Preferably use stainless steel cookware. Do not overcook your foods. Avoid or limit using the microwave oven for cooking or defrosting. Avoid heating food using soft plastic containers and plastic (cling) wrap, as they leach hormone disruptors into food that is hot, wet, fatty or acidic.

If you continue to use a microwave for reheating, cooking or defrosting, do not stand directly in front of it. Ideally move to another room when it is in use.

Food groups for Preconception Care

Proteins

Include a source of protein with every meal and every snack. This is crucial to curtail sugar cravings, help balance hormones, lose weight and improve egg quality. Proteins include the following.

Fish – ideally have three times weekly. Choose deep-sea fish high in essential fatty acids. Avoid eating farmed fish (the battery hens of the sea), large fish (e.g. tuna and shark, which may contain mercury) and crustaceans such as prawns as they are often polluted and subject to heavy metals and bacteria. Fresh fish is definitely preferable to tinned or frozen. Wild-caught salmon and sardines are good choices.

Red meats – eat organic or grass-fed red meats and in moderation. Avoid organ meats, offal (which contain high levels of pesticides) and delicatessen meats that can be high in fats, offal content, and sulphates and nitrates.

Poultry – eat only certified organically fed poultry (free range is not necessarily organic and may still be fed with hormones and antibiotics). Apart from chicken, consider other organic birds such as duck, goose, quail and turkey. Trim the skin to avoid fats.

Eggs – also choose organic. Limit their consumption only if they cause gastro-intestinal problems such as gas or constipation or other allergy symptoms.

Dairy – (if tolerant) choose organic full fat, not low fat. Do not limit to cow: try goat, sheep and buffalo. Fermented dairy such as kefir and yoghurt are easier to digest if you have digestive issues. Nut and grain milk (oat, rice, quinoa, almond) are fine as well, although not as high in protein. Avoid soy milk at all costs. The majority of soy is genetically modified and contain phytates which can block mineral absorption.

If you are **vegetarian**, you will need to combine your plant proteins to have a complete protein source. Eat nuts, grains and seeds, and legumes and pulses.

Examples include split peas, lentils, chickpeas (hummus), beans, quinoa, raw and unsalted nuts and seeds. Store nuts and seeds in the fridge, away from light and consume them within two weeks. They can be frozen. Nuts should not taste bitter.

Preparing grains and legumes

If you have digestive issues or depend on grains and legumes for a high portion of your diet, then phytates (phytic acid) could lead to mineral deficiencies. Phytic acid binds with minerals such as calcium, phosphorus, iron and zinc. This may be one of the biggest reasons why traditional societies fermented their grains. Try toasting or soaking grains, nuts and legumes before cooking.

Carbohydrates

Keep consumption of carbohydrates to moderate levels and choose low glycaemic carbohydrates where possible (mostly non-starchy vegetables, pulses and wholegrains.) Avoid high glycaemic foods (e.g. sugar, white and refined grains). Such refined carbohydrates can disrupt hormones, deplete nutrients and increase cravings. The balance of protein to carbohydrate foods should be approximately

1:1 in volume, though you can eat as much non-starchy vegetables as you like.

Aim to have:

- 80 per cent of your carbs from plants, fruit and legumes. Choose leafy greens for folate (folic acid) and iron. You can have vegetables raw; in a salad; or steamed, stir-fried or dry baked. Have no more than two pieces of fruit a day, and one cup of legumes per day (in hummus or added to salads)
- 20 per cent from wholegrains, preferably gluten-free (refer to Section 4: Chapter 18 – Going Gluten Free). Keep to one cooked cup per day
- 0 per cent from sugar!

Healthy fats

Avoid toxic non-organic saturated fats such as margarine, which disturb prostaglandin, hormone and nutrient balance. Also avoid fried fatty foods which may contribute to inflammation, such as takeaway fried chicken and fish and chips.

Stir-fries are fine. Cook with a minimal amount of sesame oil, organic butter or coconut oil. These are monounsaturated fats and will not saturate on heating. For more information on cooking with oils, see Section 4, Food Groups.

Try hummus, tahini, organic butter and/or nut butters as spread alternatives. Use cold-pressed plant-based oils on salads (extra virgin olive oil, flaxseed, nut oils). These oils are high in essential fatty acids and should not be heated. Add lemon, pepper, garlic and/or herbs to make a homemade salad dressing.

Consider cooking with duck and goose fat. These both have many health benefits and are higher in good fats than olive oil. They are semisolid at room temperature and quite heat stable. They contain approximately 35 per cent saturated fat, 52 per cent monounsaturated fat (including small amounts of antimicrobial palmitoleic acid) and about 13 per cent polyunsaturated fat. The proportion of omega-6 to omega-3 fatty acids depends on what the birds have eaten (the more grass eaten, the higher the omega-3, which is preferred). Goose fat is more like olive oil rather than butter in molecular structure. The main difference between chicken, turkey and duck fat is that duck contains more linoleic acid, while chicken and turkey contain a higher amount of polyunsaturated fats.

Spices and condiments

It is best to use salt sparingly for cooking. You may add a little sea, rock or Himalayan salt (to taste) to your prepared meal. Pepper and spices are fine to add (unless you are sensitive to them). Avoid any sauces containing sugar, salt or additives.

Beverages

Drinking two to three litres of clean, filtered water each day is recommended. Organic herbal teas aid detoxification and encourage regular bowel movements. My top choices include dandelion tea, mint tea and nettle tea.

Limit tea to one to two weak cups per day and avoid coffee, commercial fruit juice (although juicing is ok) and all soft drinks regardless if they are sugar-free (as artificial sweeteners such as aspartame is just as bad for your health). Good alternatives to tea include herb teas, fruit teas, Rooibos (caffeine-free South African tea), decaffeinated tea, or Japanese bancha (twig) tea.

Alcohol

Alcohol intake is associated with decreased fertility, even when five or fewer drinks are consumed weekly. Some studies suggest alcohol consumption can reduce your chances of conceiving by half. Alcohol is known to disrupt hormone balance, stop ovulation and interfere with conception. Therefore, it is important to avoid alcohol prior to commencing and during an IVF cycle (and when you are pregnant).

Caffeine

Caffeine can adversely affect your fertility. It's not just coffee, caffeine is also found in black tea, green tea, energy drinks and alas, chocolate.

Even decaffeinated coffee produced using the 'Swiss water method' is not recommended as the inflammatory promoting alkaloids are still present, which can contribute to uterine inflammation.

Did you know?

- More than 750mg per day of caffeine can decrease fertility by 40 per cent (to put this into perspective, a large latte can contain approximately 800mg).
- Women drinking more than three cups of coffee per day during the first trimester have an increased risk of miscarriage.
- Caffeine consumption prior to and during pregnancy is associated with prematurity, reduced foetal growth and neonatal withdrawal symptoms.

Caffeine intake linked to miscarriage

Numerous studies confirm that women who consume 200mg or more of caffeine per day (two or more cups of regular coffee or five cans of caffeinated soft drinks) have twice the miscarriage risk as women who consumed no caffeine.

The effect appears to be the caffeine itself as intake from non-coffee sources such as caffeinated soda, tea and hot chocolate showed a similar increased risk of miscarriage. Green tea and black tea also contain the same amount of caffeine as both come from the same plant.

According to the National Drug and Alcohol Research Centre at the University of New South Wales, Australia, the caffeine content of a typical 150ml cup of tea varies from 30 to 100mg, depending on how long the tea is infused and whether you brew with loose leaves (stronger) or tea bags.

In regards to coffee, the beans come in two flavours, Robusta and Arabica. Lighter-colour Robusta coffee beans contain more caffeine (2 per cent) than Arabica (1 per cent) as the roasting process removes some of the caffeine.

A typical 150ml espresso cup of coffee contains at least 90mg; drip-percolated 100-150mg and instant 60-100mg (depending on the serving spoon). What's more, whether the coffee is decaffeinated or not, it still contains chlorogenic acid which on its own or combined with caffeine has been correlated with higher homocysteine levels and inflammation.

Other sources of caffeine include cola and energy drinks. A 375ml cola drink contains approximately 40mg caffeine while a 250ml energy drink contains around 80-100mg caffeine – about the same as a shot of espresso.

Lastly, don't forget about that afternoon chocolate bar. A 30g bar has between 20 to 60mg caffeine – something worth considering when calculating a daily caffeine intake!

Smoking

Do I really have to mention smoking? Not just giving it up yourself, but also avoiding second-hand smoke wherever possible is highly recommended. Smoking can contribute to fertility issues in both men and women. In men, smoking impacts sperm counts, quality and motility. Smoking affects egg quality in women and when pregnant, her developing baby.

Cigarette smoke contains cadmium, which has an adverse effect on the production of ovarian hormones. Cotinine is another dubious ingredient in cigarette smoke which has been noted in the follicular fluid of women who are having trouble conceiving or are undergoing IVF.

Marijuana

Effects of the THC (Tetrahydrocannabinol) component from marijuana (Cannabis sativa) include hormone imbalances, irregular cycle, miscarriage, greater difficulty at delivery, increased incidence of pre-tern deliveries and abnormalities.[4]

Preconception nutritional medicine

A healthy diet is not always enough, especially in cases of significant vitamin or mineral deficiencies. Forty years of research has shown that most chronic diseases including obesity are nutrition related. Statistics reveal that although we are consuming more calories per person than ever, we seem to be receiving less nourishment.

There are key nutritional supplements that may be recommended by your doctor or naturopath such as prenatal supplements preferably containing folate as a bioactive form, probiotics, essential fatty acids and antioxidants.

Detailed information on these supplements is found in Section 5.

[4] Maccarone M. Br J Pharmacol 2008; 153:189-198

Notes

PRECONCEPTION LIFESTYLE AND STRESS SUPPORT

Fertility is a whole-body event. Preconception care isn't just about what we eat and avoiding or limiting toxins. It should also incorporate exercise, quality sleep, weight loss strategies (if appropriate) and stress management.

Exercise regularly

A varied programme of regular low-impact aerobic exercise of a minimum 30 minutes three to four times per week is recommended. Try walking, swimming and gentle jogging. Rebounding is particularly beneficial for the health of reproductive organs. Yoga is also excellent for all aspects of reproductive health.

Get adequate sleep

Sleep is restorative on so many levels – it is important to physically rest, but also to rest your mind. What's more, sleep also curbs sugar cravings and is important for hormone balance. The detoxification enzyme, glutathione, is activated during sleep, so eight hours shut-eye is critical.

Address any weight issues

One-fifth of pregnant women wanting to do IVF are clinically obese. Women with a BMI greater than 35 should lose weight prior to an IVF cycle. However, regardless of age, it is important to lose weight for many reasons. Being overweight or obese contributes to:

- Menstrual problems including lack of ovulation
- Infertility
- Miscarriage
- Impaired foetal wellbeing and increased risk of birth defects e.g. spina bifida, heart defects, cleft lip, neural tube defects

(which is not completely abolished with folate supplementation). There appears to be approximately a 7 per cent increase in the risk of birth defects for each one-unit incremental increase in BMI above 25[5]

- Problems in pregnancy such as gestational diabetes, hypertension (high blood pressure during pregnancy), pre-eclampsia and delivery complications.

Following a calorie-restricted low GL or low carbohydrate diet with good fibre levels and adequate amounts of good quality protein, along with regular exercise is recommended. For more detailed information, please refer to Section 3, Carrying Extra Weight.

Stress support

Having experienced IVF myself, I know how stressful the journey can be. Keeping stress under control leading up to and during the IVF cycle can be very difficult.

It is important to nurture and take care of yourself when preparing and going through your IVF journey. This can be done by creating a stress-support system by using tools such as visualisation, acupuncture, meditation and taking stress-supporting nutrients, herbs and flower essences. Many studies have also shown mind-body therapies can help increase IVF success rates.

Meditation and visualisation

Meditation is a wonderful way to help calm the mind and balance the body. Deep breathing reduces stress and stimulates the circulatory system. Once you have a clear mind, you feel peace and surrender to life's current circumstances, helping make your IVF journey less stressful and more peaceful.

[5] Nelson SM, Fleming RF, Hum Reprod 2007; 22(4):912-91

There are many types of meditation you can practise. For more details, please refer to Section 7, Meditation.

Ideally, practise relaxation and visualisation techniques daily. My audio *'Guided Meditation for IVF Success'* CD is a wonderful and very powerful visualisation guide for you to listen to daily and assist the relaxation process.

Emotional Freedom Technique

The theory behind Emotional Freedom Technique (EFT) is that all negative emotions are stored at a cellular level and are caused by a disruption in the body's energy system. By balancing the energy via the same system used in acupuncture (the meridians), negative emotions may be resolved, which in turn can benefit the physiological condition of a person. The release of emotions such as fear, worry and sadness gives way to rational and positive thinking. It can also generate feelings of great relief and lightness.

IVF counselling

Generally, when you begin your IVF journey, you will be put in touch with a counsellor who specialises in counselling prior and during IVF. It is a great idea to take advantage of this opportunity and have a chat. Speaking to a counsellor could help fill that gap of support that sometimes friends, and family are not able to fill or understand. Strong feelings and reactions are extremely common with IVF patients. Many patients feel much calmer and more confident after a counselling session.

You will find more detailed information on relationship support and counselling in Section 6.

Notes

Section 3

Obstacles to Overcome

This section looks at some of the common obstacles on your IVF journey and provides ways to overcome them.

Notes

STRESS AND IVF

The worse thing someone can say to you when you are embarking on an IVF cycle is 'You are too stressed. Relax and it will happen'. It is next to impossible to relax when going through the uncertainty of IVF. I know, I have been there. Negative thoughts and emotions such as guilt, worry and fear are buried in our subconscious mind and do cause stress, especially when trying for a baby. Women question everything about themselves 'Why isn't it working?' 'Is it because I did this?', 'Is it because I had a cup of coffee?'

Many couples rank infertility right up there with having a serious life-threatening disease. It is a natural tendency for human beings to want to have a child. When that ability or outcome is threatened, it can create a belief that somehow, they are not whole or not good enough or that something is seriously wrong with them.

> "Oh, what a power is motherhood, possessing
> A potent spell. All women alike
> Fight fiercely for a child."
>
> - Euripides, Iphigenia in Aulis, c. 405 B.C.

Infertility increases anxiety and pressures on relationships.

IVF is incredibly stressful – going to consultations (and sometimes having to wait hours!), waiting for scans, having numerous blood tests, hearing good news, hearing bad news, all the while trying to work and live your life. Some studies show that if women (and men) are really stressed it can affect the outcome of IVF, but the jury is still out on this, as in other studies, stress did not appear to impact IVF outcomes. How the researchers measured this, I don't know!

Despite what your specialist might say, there is ample evidence that lower stress levels mean better female and male natural fertility. Reducing stress may diminish the number of treatment cycles needed before pregnancy is obtained, may prepare the couple for an initial failure of treatment or even make the more invasive techniques unnecessary.[6]

A study cited a few years ago in the Human Reproductive Journal stated "The limited available evidence is suggestive of an association between stress and fertility, with stress having a detrimental impact on achieving a viable pregnancy through IVF treatment.[7]

The impact of stress on hormones

As a naturopath, I have been treating the impact of stress on women's hormone systems for many years. A lot of women I treat are career women. They are in their mid-30s to early 40s and usually have a well-established, successful career. This is often the same for their partner. But if their work life is stressful, this can come at a cost to their hormone health and fertility.

Adrenalin and cortisol are your body's two key stress hormones, and are closely linked: if one rises, the other follows suit. Adrenalin provides a short-term stress response and then drops quickly, while cortisol remains active and sustained for longer.

If intense stress has become a way of life, stress hormones like adrenalin and cortisol will also move to the forefront, instead of ebbing and flowing as part of the 'fight or flight' response hard-wired into us. The more of these stress hormones we have in our bloodstream, the more sensitive we become to all stimuli, not just stressful events, resulting in a persistent, constant stress state.

Adding insult to injury, an oversupply of cortisol also takes a toll on the optimal functioning of other hormones, notably your sex

[6] Camagne DM. Should fertilization treatment start with reducing stress? Hum Reprod 2006;21(7):1651-8.
[7] Ebbesen SM et. Al Stressful life events are associated with a poor in-vitro fertilization (IVF) outcome; a prospective study. Hum Reprod 2009 Sep; 24 (9): 2173-82.

hormones, oestrogen and progesterone, which in turn dampens desire and compromises fertility.

Elevated cortisol has also been implicated in inflammation, disruption of important gut bacteria, poor pelvic blood flow, thyroid health and adrenal burnout.

Progesterone can be converted into cortisol to help the body cope with the increased demands of cortisol and in some women, this depletes the progesterone available for fertility. This is called the 'cortisol steal'. Low progesterone impacts on hormone balance, cycle length and health of the endometrial (uterine) lining.

Other hormones affected by stress include prolactin, secreted from the pituitary gland, which in excess, can suppress ovulation, decrease libido and contribute to PMS symptoms. The anterior pituitary hormones, FSH and LH, are also sensitive to the impact of stress (especially in the case of hypothalamic amenorrhoea). Is it any wonder then, that stress does an impact on your IVF cycle!

Treat stress to maximise IVF success

Mind-body therapies use the power of thoughts and emotions to influence physical health. A study in *Fertility and Sterility* (an international journal for medical professionals who treat and investigate problems of infertility and human reproductive disorders) found a dramatic increase in IVF success rates for those who participated in a mind-body program prior to and during their IVF procedure.[8]

[8] Fertility & Sterility, 1 June 2011

Laughter may not be the best medicine, but it might help women's IVF success rates

A 2011 study found that women undergoing IVF treatment were more likely to become pregnant if visited by a 'medical clown' just after embryo transfer. The study was carried out on 219 women undergoing IVF at a research hospital in Israel. Results of the study indicated that women undergoing IVF treatments had a higher rate of success and becoming pregnant when they were visited by a 'medical clown' while recovering from an implantation procedure. Overall, 36 per cent became pregnant, versus 20 per cent of women who'd had a comedy-free recovery after embryo implantation.

bit.ly/hY769f Fertility and Sterility, online January 6, 2011.

Adrenal support

Stress reduction and adrenal support are crucial for women experiencing hormone problems, especially those who have luteal phase or progesterone deficiencies.

Apart from following a healthy diet, try some of these stress-relieving suggestions:

- Enjoy some daily sunlight (if possible!) and top up on vitamin D.
- Enjoy 20 minutes of evening moonlight.
- Turn off all electronic devices at least one hour before going to bed, including tablets, mobile phones and computers.
- Enjoy a candlelit bath using soy or beeswax candles which are virtually free from soot and toxins.
- Aim to get to bed no later than 10 p.m. and aim for eight hours sleep – adequate sleep is necessary for healthy hormone (in particular FSH) levels.

- Listen to your primal body. Don't overexert yourself; for example, consider yoga and walking instead of running.
- Learn to say 'no' and try not to over-commit yourself.
- To help with a positive attitude, try affirmations such as "I am making positive choices for my emotional health and wellbeing".

Your naturopath may also prescribe:

- Adrenal herbs such as Withania, Kava, Licorice, Rehmannia and Siberian ginseng
- 5 HTP (5-hydroxytryptophan) – a great nutritional supplement for anxiety (as one of my patients calls it 'water off a duck's back' remedy!)*
- SAMe (for low mood and depression)
- Magnesium, B complex and vitamin C
- Flower essences e.g. Rescue Remedy or Emergency Essence
- Theanine - a natural amino acid with relaxing and mood enhancing properties.

**Although some companies add a warning to the label to not take 5 HTP during pregnancy, this is an unsubstantiated warning and is very safe to take during the preconception months. As with all supplements and herbs recommended in this book, be guided by a qualified naturopath if this is a suitable supplement for you to take.*

For more details on supplements and herbal medicine for IVF, please refer to Section 5.

Just knowing there are options to assist with stress can be empowering.

Notes

THE AGEING FEMALE

As mentioned earlier, a woman's age is one of most important factors influencing the success of IVF when she uses her own eggs. A live birth rate of about 20 per cent for a 40-year-old woman is not quite as bad as it sounds - it's about the same chance a healthy, fertile 30-year-old woman has of becoming pregnant every month she tries, and far more than a 40-year-old woman's chance without IVF.

This is where AMH results come in. Anti-Mullerian hormone - or AMH - is a test that specialists may use to assess ovarian ageing and to measure the number of growing follicles in the ovaries (ovarian reserve); a measure, in their opinion, of fertility. Higher AMH values are thought to reflect a greater, more youthful pool of ovarian follicles and more robust fertility, whereas lower values reflect reduced fertility.

A woman's body contains millions of follicles at birth, but over time the number of follicles may decline. The levels usually peak around 24 years of age. AMH levels tend to decline as a woman transitions through peri-menopause and may be virtually undetectable after menopause.

Women with many small follicles, typical in those with PCOS, usually have higher levels of AMH and lower FSH levels. A test result of a high AMH reading may indicate PCOS and is also used to determine excessive or poor response to ovarian hyper-stimulation (caused by FSH stimulation or HCG trigger shots as part of the IVF process). Women with endometriosis tend to have low AMH levels, yet high FSH levels.

Women with low levels of AMH may also indicate low levels of follicles and immature eggs. Low levels of AMH in women under the age of 40 may also indicate Premature Ovarian Failure (POF), defined as a loss of normal ovarian function before the age of 40.

Anti-Mullerian hormone test results = chance of conception (supposedly!)

Ovarian Fertility Potential	pmol/L	ng/mL
Optimal Fertility	28.6 - 48.5	4.0 - 6.8
Satisfactory Fertility	15.7 - 28.6	2.2 - 4.0
Low Fertility	2.2 - 15.7	0.3 - 2.2
Very Low / Undetectable	0.0 - 2.2	0.0 - 0.3
High Level	> 48.5	>6.8

Many doctors use this test result to determine if you are a good candidate for IVF. It may help them determine if they should go forward with IVF or not. However, the use of this test method is still in its infancy and inaccuracies are found. In fact, one study states "caution should be exercised in the interpretation of AMH levels in the clinical setting".[9]

Issues include testing on the right day, temperature fluctuations and instability.[10] The recent use of the oral contraceptive pill (OCP) can lower AMH levels for up to three months.

However, if you have a low AMH level, there is still a chance you may fall pregnant! Many women can and do conceive both naturally and with IVF with lower AMH values, but it may take more time, and more care may be needed when selecting the kind of IVF procedure to undergo.

[9] humrep.oxfordjournals.org/content/early/2012/07/09/humrep
Oxford Journal Medicine & Health Human Reproduction Advance Access
[10] 1093/humrep/des260

How does egg health and count decline?

The good news is AMH levels are not thought to determine the quality of eggs. So how can someone with a low AMH level increase the number of follicles they have or support the health of the ones they currently have?

To begin with, eating a healthy diet, taking specific nutritional supplements and making positive lifestyle choices may be especially restorative when faced with low AMH values.

In my clinic, I continue to see AMH levels rising in women following my *'5-Step programme to increase egg health'*. One patient reported her AMH levels rising from 1.2 to 6ng/mL since following such advice. Another 33-year-old patient had an AMH reading of 1.3 and was told by her doctor she was on the verge of menopause. After just a few months of following my recommendations while waiting to commence IVF, she fell pregnant naturally. So, it seems the impossible may be possible at times!

The 5-Step programme to increase egg health

1. Address the cause

Any number of the following can contribute to a low AMH reading:

- Being overweight or obese
- Poor diet
- Smoking
- Hormone problems such as endometriosis
- Underactive thyroid gland
- Genetic mutation of 5,10-methylenetetrahydrofolate reductase (MTHFR) - involved in folate metabolism and methylation
- Immune issues such as certain autoimmune diseases
- Recent use of the oral contraceptive pill
- Environmental toxins.

2. Support the stress response

When the body is dealing with consistent, overwhelming stress, reproduction may not become the body's main focus. It is important to support the stress response.

3. Minimise toxins

Reducing exposure to toxins, even just changing to using natural cleaning products and skincare, will also contribute to improved hormone health and egg health.

4. Optimise nutrition

An egg begins as an immature follicle and goes through a maturation process from the time the ovary picks up a follicle to the ripening of the immature egg cell, called an oocyte. This oocyte is surrounded by follicular fluid and its development is related to hormone fluctuations and to the substances in this fluid, including but not limited to nutrients such as antioxidants and minerals. Therefore, improving your nutritional status can go a long way to restoring egg quality and improving your chances of IVF success.

The role of DHEA

Dehydroepiandrosterone (DHEA) is a hormone that has been proven to raise levels of AMH and improve ovarian reserve.

When AMH levels are low, IVF success rates tend to suffer compared to success rates of women with higher levels of AMH - which indicate a better quality of ovarian reserve. But when DHEA is supplemented in women with poor ovarian reserve prior to IVF, embryo quality and pregnancy rates increase.[11]

In a study of 120 women with diminished ovarian reserve, the control group were supplemented with 25mg of DHEA three times a day for 30 to 120 days. AMH levels were found to significantly

[11] J Assisted Reprod Genet. 2007 Dec;24(12):629-34. Epub 2007 Dec 11. Update on the use of dehydroepiandrosterone supplementation among women with diminished ovarian function. Barad D., et al.

improve after treatment with DHEA, especially in women under 38 years of age, compared to no change with the placebo group.[12]

If you choose to take DHEA, be sure to check with your doctor and naturopath, who can prescribe a quality, pharmaceutical-grade DHEA.

DHEA may be one of the most powerful ovary-rejuvenating supplements to date.

5. Make appropriate exercise and lifestyle changes

Ensuring you maintain a regular exercise routine (nothing too strenuous) and getting eight hours of quality sleep each night are also important factors for optimising egg health.

So, the next time you think "time is running out", just pause, take a deep breath and replace such thoughts with the mantra "I am doing everything I possibly can to become pregnant".

Remember, you are taking positive steps to optimise your health and your fertility such as eating well, minimising toxins, exercising, taking specific supplements for your situation and implementing stress management strategies.

Feel reassured you are doing everything you can to maximise your chances of IVF success.

[12] Reprod Biomed Online. 2010 Sep;21(3):360-5. Epub 2010 Apr 18. Improvement in diminished ovarian reserve after dehydroepiandrosterone supplementation. Gleicher N, et al.

Notes

CARRYING EXTRA WEIGHT

The prevalence of obesity is increasing at an alarming rate. In the UK (and no doubt many other countries), obesity affects one-fifth of the female population and approximately 20 per cent of women of reproductive age. In addition, one-fifth of pregnant women booking for antenatal care are clinically obese.

Being overweight, particularly visceral obesity (belly fat), contributes to:

- Menstrual problems including PCOS and lack of ovulation
- Syndrome X/metabolic syndrome, which causes blood sugar imbalances, insulin resistance, raised cholesterol levels, and can lead to diabetes and heart disease
- Infertility
- Miscarriage
- Complications in pregnancy such as gestational diabetes, high blood pressure, pre-eclampsia and delivery complications
- An increased risk of babies being born with abnormalities e.g. spina bifida, heart defects and cleft lip.

Fact: You can increase your chances of IVF success if you can reach a healthy weight before you have treatment. IVF is more likely to be successful if your body mass index (BMI) is between 19 and 30.

Dieting during pregnancy is not always recommended, so now is a great time to start making healthy eating choices that you can stick to once you conceive.

Talk to your doctor and naturopath/nutritionist if you need advice about changing your diet or starting exercise. Ideally aim to lose 1kg (2lb) a week.

Some weight loss tips...

Eat breakfast every day

You're less likely to snack on unhealthy foods later if you have a bowl of porridge with some ground flaxseeds, almond, sunflower and pumpkin seeds; or two poached eggs with some tomato and avocado first thing in the morning.

Watch your portion sizes

Keep an eye on your portion sizes at mealtimes. Eat from a smaller plate if it helps.

Cut out all forms of sugar

That means no chocolate, cakes, biscuits, doughnuts, dried fruit, jam and fruit juice.

Eat the right types of carbs

Aim to consume most of your carbohydrates from vegetables, fruit and just a small amount of grain. Suitable quantities per serve include:

- 1 cup cooked vegetables or 2 cups salad vegetables, maximum 2 serves of low GI fruit per day e.g. 1 apple and 1 cup melon, and limited grains including (preferably gluten-free) 1 slice of bread, and 1/3 cup of cooked rice, pasta or noodles.

Adding grains to your meals is optional and by limiting or leaving grains out, your weight loss will be greater. However, it is important to remember complex carbohydrates contain beneficial fibre, which is important for healthy digestion and bowel regularity, healthy cholesterol levels, healthy blood sugar levels and greater satiety.

Have healthy snacks

Choose healthy snacks such as a handful of fresh fruit and nuts, a homemade protein ball or some hummus on two oat cakes. That way you won't succumb to high or refined sugar options when you're out or at work.

Include protein

Ensure you include adequate protein as part of every meal and snack. Sources include lean red meat, organic/free-range poultry, eggs, seafood and shellfish, legumes, lentils, protein powders, nuts and seeds. Protein helps to stabilise your blood sugar levels and keeps you feeling satisfied for longer. You will notice a decrease in sugar cravings within about two weeks when you incorporate protein into every meal including snacks.

Don't forget good fats

Good fats are essential for hormone production, thyroid gland health, cell quality, skin health, heart health and cognitive function. Omega 3 Essential Fatty Acids (EFAs) include oily fish such as herring, mackerel, mullet, salmon and sardines. Other sources of good fat include coconut oil, flaxseed oil, krill oil, avocados, nuts and seeds.

Start exercising

Exercise is important, too. If you build it into your daily routine, perhaps walking briskly to work, getting off the bus one stop earlier, or taking the stairs, it will be more achievable. Some people are motivated to move more by using a pedometer or wearing a Fitbit fitness tracker. The goal is to achieve 20,000 steps each day. Joining a group can help motivate you to lose weight and keep it off. You'll be offered regular advice on exercise and diet, as well as support from others.

Extreme weight loss from crash-dieting can deplete your body's nutritional stores. Losing weight gradually through healthy eating and regular exercise is the best option. Long-term lifestyle changes are more successful than quick-fix approaches.

Recipes for homemade protein balls, chia seed puddings and delicious, nutritious weight-loss smoothies can be found in the companion '*The IVF Diet Cookbook*'.

Weight gain and PCOS

If you have weight gain associated with PCOS, by losing weight it is possible to resume regular menstrual cycles with regular ovulation and improve your chances of conception and pregnancy. Even losing a mere 5 per cent of your weight increases pregnancy rates in women with PCOS.[13]

Great weight loss advice can be found in my book, *'The Natural PCOS Diet'*. (www.jennyblondel.com)

[13] Crosignani PG, et al. Overweight and obese anovulatory patients with polycystic ovaries: parallel improvements in anthropometric indices, ovarian physiology and fertility rate induced by diet. Hum Reprod. 2003 Sep;18(9):1928-32.

THYROID GLAND PROBLEMS

If you came to me for help with an irregular menstrual cycle, infertility and IVF support, I would think very carefully about your thyroid. It wouldn't matter if you already had another diagnosis such as PCOS or hypothalamic amenorrhoea. It wouldn't matter if your doctor had said at some point that your thyroid is normal. I would still consider your thyroid health. Why? Because insufficient thyroid hormone production and autoimmune diseases of the thyroid gland can be a common reason for infertility and IVF failure.

A robust thyroid gland is necessary for optimal fertility.

> Research published in the *Obstetrician & Gynaecologist* journal proves the long-suspected theory that thyroid disorders can contribute to ovulation, fertility and pregnancy problems, and recommends that women having trouble conceiving be tested for an over or underactive thyroid. While people who have chronic thyroid problems will experience obvious symptoms, undiagnosed hypothyroidism can have effects on fertility as well.
>
> A Jefferys, M Vanderpump, E Yasmin. **Thyroid dysfunction and reproductive health.** The Obstetrician & Gynaecologist, January 2015 DOI: 10.1111/tog.12161

The thyroid gland is located at the front of the throat alongside the voice box. Every cell in the body depends on the thyroid to regulate a wide range of metabolic processes.

The thyroid gland is important for maintaining healthy weight and metabolism, mood health, energy, circulation, digestion health, fertility (necessary for healthy ovulation), skin and hair health.

An underactive thyroid gland can result in a variety of symptoms including infertility, unexplained weight gain, low mood, cold hands and feet, constipation and fatigue, to name just a few.

Thyroid health is dependent on key thyroid hormone activity. Thyroid releasing hormone (TRH) is released from the hypothalamus located within the brain. TRH stimulates the pituitary gland at the base of the brain to release thyroid stimulating hormone (TSH), which in turn stimulates the thyroid gland to produce thyroxine (T4) and triiodothyronine (T3).

The majority of T4 is converted to more active T3 in the liver. Thyroid hormones are manufactured using iodine and the amino acid tyrosine which the body sources from dietary protein. The conversion of T4 to T3 is assisted by adequate dietary intake of two critical minerals – zinc and selenium.

Thyroid health is important for mums-to-be for two key reasons:

- A healthy thyroid aids normal growth and development of the unborn baby. The thyroid hormones fuel healthy nervous system development. In fact, low thyroid hormone activity is linked to intellectual delays in infants and children.
- Your thyroid is central to a healthy pregnancy. A drop in thyroid hormone activity during pregnancy can make you more prone to fatigue, hair loss, mood changes, morning sickness and other complications.

  Low body temperature can also affect the foetus as the rapidly dividing cells of the developing baby require a precise temperature range for ongoing division to take place. When your body temperature is too low, the developing baby may be unable to continue to grow. This also increases the risk of early miscarriage.

Factors contributing to Thyroid Imbalance

Below are the main factors that put you at risk of developing a thyroid problem:

- Stress is one of the major driving factors contributing to a thyroid gland problem. Stress affects your body's natural balance and can have significant consequences on your hormone balance, digestion, immune system function, mood and vitality. Elevated cortisol has a direct impact on thyroid health as it can lead to decreased T3 levels and subsequent ovulation problems; increased levels of reverse T3; and increased risk of autoimmune thyroid disease.

- Adrenal fatigue due to long-term stress. Adrenal fatigue often goes hand-in-hand with an underactive thyroid. It is next to impossible to successfully recover from a thyroid disorder when you have a co-existing adrenal problem. It is important to support adrenal health to prevent and treat any adrenal dysfunction.

- Poor liver function. Your liver plays an important role in thyroid hormone metabolism. It is one of the main sites where conversion of T4 to T3 takes place. Your liver also supports ongoing detoxification.

- Active or latent infections e.g. Epstein Barr virus.

- Gluten and other food intolerance (especially dairy and soy).

- Specific mineral deficiencies. This includes low body stores of iodine, zinc and selenium.

- Exposure to hormone disrupting chemicals such as phthalates, PCBs, BPA, dioxins and bromides (such as high fluoride in water sources), as well as exposure to environmental toxins. This includes pesticides and industrial chemicals. Thyroid problems are becoming more common as we experience greater exposure to environmental chemicals and pollution.

- Heavy metal toxicity. Sources include mercury from dental fillings and old lead paints.

- Genetic susceptibility. Thyroid disorders tend to run in families. If your family has any type of autoimmune illness, you also have a greater risk of developing a thyroid problem.

- Exposure to low-level electromagnetic radiation (EMR) from mobile phones, microwave ovens and Wi-Fi devices can zap your thyroid. Research has already established that the electromagnetic fields emitted by mobile phones may cause detrimental effects on thyroid function.

- Acute exposure to radiation or radioactive fallout.

- Candidiasis. A candida overgrowth in the digestive tract is usually associated with a systemic yeast infection in the rest of the body. This can weaken your immunity and undermine your overall health and vitality.

- Other hormone imbalances.

Thyroid testing

A single TSH test is widely considered by doctors to be the medical 'gold standard' when assessing thyroid health. TSH is the messenger hormone that signals the thyroid to produce the two main thyroid hormones T4 and T3.

But for many people with an underactive thyroid, the body is not properly converting T4 to T3. So it also makes sense to test T4 and T3 levels. When you test for these hormones, it can reveal if the thyroid gland is producing adequate T4 and that the T4 is converting sufficient levels of the more potent T3.

T3 provides the best clue as to how your thyroid is working as it is the more active thyroid hormone to help 'rev' up your body. T3 is necessary for ovulation, assists energy metabolism and weight loss, and protects against heart palpitations. Low T3 levels are associated with sluggish metabolism and many of the indicators of an underactive thyroid.

If your T3 levels are low, I suggest requesting a reverse T3 test to find out if your body is producing an active or inactive form of T3. Reverse T3 slows metabolism and when reverse T3 levels get too high, it sparks many of the signs and symptoms normally associated with an underactive thyroid.

Find out your TSH reading

You may be told your thyroid is fine when your TSH test result falls within the 'normal' range. However, a TSH reading within the established reference range can be misleading and does not automatically rule out a low thyroid issue.

There are also questions about what level should be considered normal and the logic of using a very wide reference range. Current research shows TSH between 0.5 and 2.0 mIU/L is ideal. A TSH level greater than 2.5 mIU/L is a sign of hypothyroidism. For peak fertility and miscarriage prevention, the reading should be closer to the 1.3 to 1.5 range.

More than just TSH should be tested to properly investigate your thyroid health.

Why test thyroid antibodies?

Testing for thyroid antibody levels can screen for possible autoimmune activity within the thyroid. This test measures if there is an autoimmune attack on your thyroid. Autoimmune thyroid disease is the most common type of thyroid disease in developed countries.

A positive test for thyroid antibodies is strong evidence that thyroid disease may well be contributing to your fertility problems. Highly elevated levels of thyroid antibodies are commonly associated with Hashimoto's thyroiditis. In fact, Hashimoto's thyroiditis is the leading cause of hypothyroidism particularly in women.[14] A single TSH test will fail to uncover this common thyroid disorder.

In women undergoing IVF, the presence of thyroid antibodies combined with a high TSH reading (reflecting an underactive thyroid) increases the risk of implantation failure and unsuccessful pregnancy. The message here: always make sure your doctor checks for thyroid antibodies. If they are present, IVF patients are often treated with intravenous immune globulin before the embryo transfer.

> If you suspect your thyroid gland many not be functioning properly, ask your doctor and/or naturopath for a full thyroid panel - TSH, T4, T3, reverse T3 and thyroid antibodies.

Lastly, ask your doctor to consider your family history. If you have a direct family member (mother or sister) with thyroid disease, then you are at risk, and you should qualify for further investigation.

How to treat thyroid gland problems

- Address the cause. Find out from your doctor and/or naturopath why your thyroid gland is not balanced.
- Your doctor may prescribe thyroxine treatment or compounded T4/slow release T3.
- Eliminate gluten from your diet to reduce thyroid autoimmunity.
- Maintain healthy intestinal bacteria to reduce thyroid autoimmunity.

[14] Australian Thyroid Foundation

- Incorporate dietary sources of iodine from sea vegetables and seafood.
- Your naturopath may prescribe herbal medicine such as Bladderwrack (great source of iodine), Withania and Bacopa to help maintain healthy thyroid function.

Top nutrients to assist thyroid health

Iodine

Iodine is an essential component of T4 and T3. The three and four indicate the number of iodine molecules contained within the thyroid hormone. Low iodine intake has become a common cause of thyroid health problems.

The thyroid selectively concentrates iodine in amounts necessary to support ongoing production of the thyroid hormones. The body is not able to make iodine so a steady supply from dietary sources is necessary. Since much of the world's iodine is found in the ocean, the leading dietary sources include sea vegetables and seafood.

Iodine supplements are effective for preventing and treating an iodine deficiency and are generally considered safe when taken as recommended. A daily dose of iodine from an iodine supplement must not exceed 300 micrograms per day, unless otherwise prescribed by your doctor or naturopath. High doses (>1mg) of iodine can be harmful, so please be careful (especially if you are deficient in selenium).

Zinc

This mineral assists conversion of T4 to the more active T3, required for metabolism. Adequate T3 activity helps reduce many of the symptoms commonly associated with an underactive thyroid. A daily dose between 20-40mg elemental zinc per day may be recommended by your doctor or naturopath.

Selenium

Did you know that after iodine the next nutrient to concentrate in the thyroid is selenium? In fact, the thyroid has the highest concentration of selenium compared to any other organ in the body.

Selenium teams up with zinc to assist ongoing conversion of T4 to T3. It also helps protect the thyroid from damage due to autoimmune disorders such as Hashimoto's thyroiditis. A daily dose may vary from 100 to 400mcg per day. Once again, be guided by your naturopath or doctor.

Inositol

In women with autoimmune hypothyroiditis, supplemental inositol reduces TSH to physiological levels and works synergistically with selenium to reduce auto-antibodies by almost 50%.

B group vitamins

These vitamins help maintain healthy function of the nervous system and assist energy metabolism. The body experiences an increased demand for B group vitamins during periods of stress, making regular intake necessary for most people!

Vitamin B6 can be particularly useful to help manage low moods commonly associated with a thyroid gland problem. Pyridoxal 5'-phosphate (P5P) is considered a superior form to aid mood as this is the active form of B6. A daily dose of 25mg in this form twice daily may be recommended.

Need IVF because of PCOS?

You may have a thyroid problem too. If you are embarking on the IVF journey because you have PCOS, there is an increased likelihood that you may also have an underactive thyroid or even a thyroid autoimmune disease. Just having a diagnosis of PCOS triples the risk for having thyroid autoimmune disease, which can

exacerbate infertility and greatly increase miscarriage rates if left undiagnosed and untreated.
A number of studies have identified a link between PCOS and increased incidence of autoimmune thyroid disease. Sadly, doctors still do not automatically test women with PCOS to see if they have elevated levels of thyroid auto-antibodies which could elevate risks for miscarriage and IVF failure.

A 2013 Italian study cited in the *European Journal of Obstetrics, Gynaecology and Reproductive Biology* tested for thyroid autoimmune disease in 113 women with PCOS and discovered that 27 per cent had the disease. In addition, 43 per cent of the women had subclinical hypothyroidism, which is also linked with increased miscarriage risks if undiagnosed and untreated. The outcome of this study suggests that PCOS patients should be screened for autoimmune thyroid disease.[15]

A German study also sought to discover the relationship between PCOS and autoimmune thyroid disease; over 30 months the researchers examined the thyroids of 175 women with PCOS along with 168 age-matched controls.[16]

The women with PCOS had significantly more (26.9 per cent) cases of elevated thyroid antibodies than the controls (8.3 per cent). Ultrasound findings also revealed that 42.3 per cent of PCOS women had thyroid tissue changes consistent with thyroid autoimmune disease and 10 per cent of PCOS women had out-of-range TSH levels compared with only 1.8 per cent of controls. This led the researchers to conclude that patients with PCOS have a threefold higher prevalence of thyroid autoimmune disease.

[15] Garelli S, Masiero S, Plebani M, Chen S, Furmaniak J, Armanini D, Betterle C.: Eur J Obstet Gyne Reprod Biol. 2013 Mar 30. pii: S0301-2115(13)00116-4. doi: 10.1016/j.ejogrb.2013.03.003. [Epub ahead of print] High prevalence of chronic thyroiditis in patients with polycystic ovary syndrome.

[16] Eur J Endocrinol. 2004 Mar;150(3):363-9. High prevalence of autoimmune thyroiditis in patients with polycystic ovary syndrome. Jannsen OE, Mehlmauer N, Hahn S, Offner AH, Gartner R. German

In summary

If you have PCOS make sure that you have a comprehensive thyroid test including thyroid antibodies. If the TSH reading is high, your doctor may also request a thyroid ultrasound, which can pick up early thyroid autoimmune disease before antibodies become manifest in the blood.

PCOS AND INFERTILITY

Polycystic Ovarian Syndrome (PCOS) is an endocrine disorder that causes fertility problems, weight gain, insulin resistance, menstrual problems, acne, hair loss, and hirsutism. Not all women with PCOS have these signs and symptoms nor do all have PCOS ovaries either. Conversely, not all women with these signs and symptoms have PCOS. The so-called cysts are just one of the many signs and symptoms of PCOS. The lack of ovulation associated with PCOS is the leading cause of infertility in women of reproductive age.

A Poly-glandular Syndrome

Polycystic ovarian syndrome is not actually an ovarian condition, it is far more than just a reproductive problem – it affects an entire cascade of hormones and each PCOS sufferer's experience with this syndrome is very different. There are ovarian consequences, but the pathophysiology is not ovarian in origin. Hormones are the problem. Ovaries are the victim.

The Hypothalamic-Pituitary-Adrenal (HPA) axis, thyroid gland, pancreas and the liver are usually implicated in this syndrome. Because PCOS can affect a women's appearance, metabolism and fertility, many psychological issues such as anxiety, depression, relationship problems and eating disorders can manifest.

Signs and Symptoms of PCOS

The cysts on polycystic ovaries are tiny and look like black dots on the ovary on an ultrasound. The cysts are actually multiple immature ova (eggs that have failed to fully mature) that have not been released from the ovary.

A polycystic ovary has, by definition, more than 12 small undeveloped follicles compared to a normal ovary averaging 6 to 12 variously sized follicles.

But why are the follicles tiny? Because ovulation did not occur that month. An ultrasound cannot explain why ovulation did not occur, nor can it predict whether ovulation will occur the next month. Sometimes ovulation just doesn't happen, and that's why normal women have polycystic ovaries 25 percent of the time. That's why experts now agree that PCOS cannot be diagnosed by ultrasound.

Signs and symptoms of PCOS may include:

- infertility
- ovarian/pelvic pain
- irregular or absent menstruation
- irregular or absent ovulation
- increased facial and body hair (hirsutism) and/or male pattern hair growth
- weight gain and obesity especially around the trunk (apple or android body shape, especially after age of 30)
- acne, oily skin and increased skin pigmentation, skin tags
- hyperkeratosis of the skin
- reduced libido
- fatigue (may be a result of sleep apnoea)
- hypoglycaemic episodes
- mood swings/depression
- hypothyroidism
- hyperprolactinaemia

You may only experience a few of these symptoms or may be able to tick them all.

Causes of PCOS

While researchers are not certain of the exact cause of PCOS, it is known that an imbalance of the endocrine system is responsible for many of the changes associated with PCOS. It can be difficult to say where it starts. Hormonal imbalance, stress, thyroid gland problems, and genetics play a role. Immediate female relatives of women with PCOS (i.e. daughters or sisters) have up to a 50% chance of having this condition.

In addition, if we look at the different types of PCOS, this too, gives us more understanding as to potential causes of PCOS.

1) Insulin-Resistant PCOS

Insulin resistance is the hallmark condition of our modern age, affecting 1 in 4 adults. This is the classic type of PCOS and by far the most common, affecting 50-70% of PCOS-sufferers. High insulin and leptin impede ovulation and stimulate the ovaries to make more androgen such as testosterone. Insulin resistance can be caused by poor diet, stress (DHEA, an adrenal hormone is found to be elevated in 50% of women with PCOS – contributing to elevated androgens), leptin resistance, smoking, trans fats, environmental toxins such as Bisphenol-A (BPA) and the pill. Sufferers may be of normal weight or overweight.

2) Pill-Induced PCOS or Post-Pill PCOS

It is known that the pill can also contribute to insulin resistance, which in turn, contributes to PCOS. It can also lead to weight gain, suppresses thyroid function, increases the likelihood of depression and the deposition of cellulite. The pill can also suppress the pituitary-ovarian communication, which of course it's designed to do, but that suppression is supposed to be temporary. Unfortunately, when some women stop taking the pill, they experience an ongoing elevation of Luteinising hormone (LH), a pituitary hormone which is elevated in PCOS patients, contributing to the many symptoms, including amenorrhea.

3) Inflammatory PCOS

As we know, insulin resistance is a significant contributor to weight gain and the more weight a woman carries, the more inflammatory markers she will make. However, these levels are increased not only in overweight women with PCOS but also in healthy weight women with PCOS. Increased inflammatory markers found in PCOS patients can be as a result of stress, environmental toxins, intestinal permeability and inflammatory foods such as gluten or A1 casein from dairy. Inflammation is a problem for PCOS because it impedes ovulation, disrupts hormone receptors, and stimulates adrenal androgens such DHEA and androstenedione.

4) Hidden-Cause PCOS

This is least complex type of PCOS. Frequently I encounter a PCOS patient who does not meet any of the criteria for the first 3 types of PCOS. Usually there is one single cause blocking ovulation. Once that single cause is addressed, this type of PCOS often resolves quickly, usually within 3-4 months. Common hidden causes of PCOS include:

- too much soy - can block ovulation in some women
- gluten intolerance – up to 85% of PCOS sufferers have gluten sensitivity
- thyroid dysfunction - the ovaries need T3 thyroid hormone for ovulation to occur
- vegetarian diet – can contribute to a zinc deficiency, and the ovaries need zinc
- iodine deficiency - the ovaries require iodine (caution with iodine supplementation)
- artificial sweeteners - impair insulin and leptin signalling
- too little starch in the diet – hormones need the right balance of the right type of carbohydrates
- exposure to xenoestrogens (environmental oestrogens)

NB. It is important to acknowledge there will be some overlap between these 4 types. For example, inflammation is a major cause of both insulin resistance and thyroid disease (Types 1, 3, and 4).

In summary

Some of the causes discussed here may also be consequences of PCOS. In other words, we have an amazingly complex network of interacting variables, each of which influences the other. PCOS is not a simple condition with a single cause.

Renaming PCOS

So why is this condition called PCOS?

In July 2016 a new name for the condition was proposed: **Metabolic Reproductive Syndrome.** Dr. Robert A. Rizza from the Mayo Clinic sums up the name change: 'The name PCOS focuses on criteria – namely the polycystic ovarian morphology – that is neither necessary nor sufficient to diagnose the syndrome. It is time to assign a name that reflects the complex metabolic, hypothalamic, pituitary, ovarian, and adrenal interactions that characterise PCOS.

Dietary Considerations for PCOS

Losing excess weight and controlling inflammation cannot be emphasised enough. If you have PCOS and are overweight, losing even just 5-10% of your body weight may resume regular ovulation.

Following a low carbohydrate diet balanced with adequate protein and good fats is recommended if you need to lose weight. Most of my PCOS patients are also advised to avoid dairy and gluten.

In addition, cut out sugar, high fructose syrups (including dates, and honey, and maple syrup) and refined carbohydrates. Also consider intermittent fasting.

Conversely, underweight women with PCOS need to ensure they are eating enough food. The glucose-sensitive receptors in the hypothalamus require a certain level of carbohydrate in the diet to trigger ovulation – the 'ovarian set point' (which can be different for every woman). Following a 'low carbohydrate diet' can contribute to amenorrhoea so if you are underweight, incorporate more complex carbohydrates including brown rice, potato, or sweet potato every night for three months to activate ovarian signalling.

The following general dietary recommendations are important for women with PCOS:

- The brassica family contain several powerful nutrients that help metabolise oestrogen (Indole-3 acetate, indole-3 carbonyl, diindolylmethane, sulforaphane and phenyl isothiocyanates) to enhance liver detoxification processes. Broccoli and kale sprouts are especially potent.
- The alliums, including garlic, onions, scallions, chives and leeks, are rich in sulphur-containing amino acids and the powerful flavone anti-oxidant quercetin. These compounds help the liver detoxify and reduce the production of oestrogen.
- A few grams a day of seaweed influences nutritional and hormonal pathways to help reduce a sluggish metabolism and feed the endocrine system.
- Phytoestrogens are plant compounds with structural features similar to endogenous oestrogen. However, because they are weaker, they can act as partial agonists. Lentils are a good source of phytoestrogens. Two tablespoons daily of freshly-ground flaxseed delivers a high lignan content assisting a healthy oestrogen balance.
- Mushrooms (such as shitake and reishi) regulate aromatase and regulate oestrogen levels and may be used to manage various hormone related pathologies as well as helping to stabilise the HPA (adrenal) axis.
- Spearmint tea, and Apigenin, a flavone found in chamomile and green tea can help reduce symptoms of androgen excess and assist ovulation.

Naturopathic Recommendations

The following supplements may be recommended by your naturopath or healthcare professional:

- Detoxification formulas to facilitate healthy oestrogen metabolism and removal such as calcium d-glucarate
- Magnesium for its anti-inflammatory, insulin control and adrenal support
- B vitamins, namely B1, B6, B12 for hormone regulation, methylation and histamine balance
- Chromium for blood sugar regulation and insulin responsiveness
- Inositol which increases ovulation and cycle regularity; decreases total testosterone and improves insulin resistance, dose range 4-10g/day
- Quercetin to reduce histamine release and inflammation 600mg-2g/day
- Vitamin D if deficient - 3x oral treatments of 50,000iu every 20 days/10,000iu/day for 8 weeks
- Iodine helps to resolve cysts (with the herb thuja) and is beneficial for thyroid health if deficient (dose with caution)
- Selenium, an antioxidant is also indicated for thyroid dysfunction
- Zinc is anti-inflammatory, antioxidant, is a natural aromatase inhibitor; indicated for insulin resistance, intestinal permeability; and mood support (anxiety)
- Omega 3 fish oils decrease total cholesterol and improves insulin resistance
- Alpha Lipoic acid, a potent antioxidant, improves insulin's responsiveness
- N-acetyl Cysteine (NAC) increases ovulation and pregnancy rate in PCOS (1200-1800 mg/day)
- Resveratrol, an antioxidant polyphenol found in red wine and red grapes, reduces ovarian androgen production and inhibit leptin secretion from fat cells.

- SAMe - considering the role methylation plays in both histamine degradation and oestrogen metabolism, supporting healthy SAMe synthesis may be useful, particularly if depression is a symptom
- DIM (diindolylmethane), a phytonutrient derived from cruciferous vegetables, has a positive influence on oestrogen metabolism and is a natural aromatase inhibitor. It is effective for acne and hirsutism.
- Probiotics – to re-establish a healthy gut microbiome

Herbal medicine

A recent study using a herbal preparation of licorice, peony, St john's wort and cinnamon for 3 months demonstrated weight loss around stomach: decrease of LH, increase in energy, improved fasting insulin and quality of life and increased pregnancy rate. https://www.ncbi.nlm.nih.gov/pmc/articles/PMC4528347/

Additional herbs that may be indicated for PCOS include Black cohosh, Tribulus terrestis, Saw palmetto, Vitex agnus castus (chaste tree), Thuja, and Berberine containing herbs which have been demonstrated to be as effective as metformin for insulin resistance.

https://www.ncbi.nlm.nih.gov/pmc/articles/PMC5839379/

Lifestyle

- Exercise, preferably in the morning, is a must for your PCOS patients. Weight resistance especially thighs/legs assists with insulin resistance and weigh loss.
- Reduce stress and exposure to environmental toxins like pesticides and plastics.
- Quit smoking – book your patient in for the Bicom 'Stop Smoking' therapy.
- Get eight hours sleep (ideally unbroken).
- Castor oil packs for 'cysts', 3-4 x weekly.

INFLAMMATION

When most people hear the word 'inflammation', they think of a swollen ankle, red and irritated eyes, or the pain of an injury. This is called acute inflammation, which occurs over a short period of time and is a helpful process in the body in response to any sort of trauma or injury. This type of inflammation helps to promote healing and prevent infection.

On the other hand, prolonged or chronic, often unseen internal inflammation is harmful and associated with many female reproductive issues including infertility, recurrent miscarriage, PCOS, endometriosis, thyroid gland problems, pelvic inflammatory disease (PID), Type II diabetes, heart disease and autoimmune disorders.

In autoimmune disorders, the body produces antibodies that attack healthy tissue, causing inflammation. Examples contributing to infertility include autoimmune-induced miscarriage, antisperm antibodies and Hashimoto's thyroiditis.

A note on histamine

I always test histamine levels for all my fertility patients. Why? Interestingly, here we can have a 'chicken or egg' scenario. Higher levels of oestrogen promote histamine release, while histamine elevations are also believed to increase oestrogen. During the menstrual cycle, histamine is higher in the oestrogen-driven stages and lower in the progesterone-dominant stages. Environmental oestrogens (e.g. xenoestrogens such as BPA) can also promote greater histamine release.

Histamine also appears to play a role in ovulation. High levels of histamine promote inflammation are observed in women with PCOS (also pelvic adhesions e.g. endometriosis). It is thought that this may impact ovulation and compromise fertility.

Following a low-histamine diet or at least reducing amines in the diet can assist with elevated histamine and thereby inflammation.

How to control inflammation

In regards to fertility, losing excess weight and controlling inflammation cannot be emphasised enough. Any woman wanting to optimise her reproductive health, or recover from a reproductive health issue, should eat a low acid/alkaline diet rich in anti-inflammatory foods.

Many foods consumed daily have been shown to contribute to chronic inflammation. Processed, refined foods (which are acidic) should be substituted for alkaline whole foods – this is the foundation for promoting healthy inflammatory response. In addition, there are specific foods that naturally inhibit inflammation.

Top 5 anti-inflammatory foods

1. Salmon

This cold-water fish is high in the omega-3 essential fatty acids DHA (docosahexaenoic acid) and EPA (eicosapentaenoic acid). DHA and EPA are both anti-inflammatory. Aim to eat salmon at least two times per week, or substitute with other cold-water fish such as mackerel, sardines or trout.

2. Pineapple

This fruit contains bromelain, a protease plant enzyme, found in the core of pineapples. Bromelain is anti-inflammatory and has been shown to increase cervical mucous and is reported to improve uterine lining quality (refer to Section 4, Dietary Guidelines for Each Stage of the IVF Cycle).

Consume pineapple three to five times weekly, with some of the core still intact. Pineapple is excellent in smoothies with mint and some fresh ginger root. Make sure the pineapple is fresh or frozen, rather than canned.

3. Garlic, ginger and turmeric

Garlic, ginger and especially turmeric are anti-inflammatory as well as immune boosting. Lavishly add all of these to your cooking!

Add fresh sliced garlic to homemade salad dressings, nut dips, soups, stir-fries and casseroles.

Freshly grated or sliced ginger is warming and healing. Try adding one-inch square of peeled fresh ginger root to a fresh juice blend or infuse as a tea. Ginger also supports healthy digestion, one of the first steps to healing inflammatory diseases.

Turmeric is the yellow spice containing curcumin, a powerful anti-inflammatory plant chemical. Add to stir-fries, curry dishes, brown rice dishes, casseroles and soups.

4. Flaxseeds

High in fibre and essential fatty acids, flaxseed is excellent for helping reduce chronic inflammation. The high fibre content also protects the gut from absorbing inflammatory toxins. They also promote healthy oestrogen metabolism.

It is best to eat these health-promoting seeds freshly ground to receive the full benefits. The body cannot digest the whole seed, whereas ground flaxseeds are digested easily and assist in healthy stool formulation. Store the ground flaxseed in an airtight container in the refrigerator. Have two tablespoons daily. Add to meals, smoothies, homemade granola/muesli or porridge.

5. Dark leafy green vegetables

Dark leafy green vegetables such as seaweed, collard greens, Swiss chard, broccoli and spinach are not only alkalising but high in antioxidants such as vitamins C and E, as well as fibre and phytonutrients. Vitamin E in particular protects the body from pro-inflammatory molecules known as cytokines. Be sure to lightly steam them, as this improves the bioavailability of the nutrients, while also helping to maintain a healthy gastrointestinal mucosa. Try to eat one to two servings of at least one of these vegetables daily, either in a green smoothie (blanched first), salad or as a side dish of vegetables.

Notes

HIGH HOMOCYSTEINE LEVELS

Elevated levels of homocysteine can contribute to IVF failure and miscarriage.

What is homocysteine?

Homocysteine is an amino acid produced by the body, usually as a by-product of eating animal protein. However, prescription drugs, smoking, coffee, alcohol, high dairy intake, obesity, age, and gene mutations can all contribute to elevated homocysteine levels. High homocysteine levels have been linked to miscarriage, IVF failure, heart disease, stroke, macular degeneration, hearing loss, migraine, brain atrophy, dementia and cancer. Researchers believe homocysteine affects the heart by damaging the blood vessel lining and promoting blood clot formation.

The implications for women and fertility

Studies have confirmed elevated homocysteine levels in the follicular fluid of women having difficulty getting pregnant naturally or with IVF procedures. High levels are also associated with poor embryo quality.[17] Follicles exposed to low levels of homocysteine is associated with a better embryo quality and a higher degree of maturity.

Studies have also shown blood clots were strongly associated with women older than 39 who underwent IVF and had elevated homocysteine levels.

Other articles confirm that elevated homocysteine levels are present in women who miscarry – more so if they also have a MTHFR gene mutation (see the next chapter) contributing to folate metabolism errors and problems with methylation.

[17] Boxmeer JC et.al IVF outcomes are associated with biomarkers of the homocysteine pathway in monofollicular fluid. Hum. Reprod. 2009 May; 24(5):1059-66.

Elevated homocysteine levels have also been associated with clotting issues such as antiphospholipid antibodies and Factor V Leiden.

In addition, elevated homocysteine has also been correlated with gestational diabetes and pre-eclampsia during pregnancy. It is also associated with placenta problems and birth defects including neural tube defects, heart malformations and cleft lip.

There is even some research that supports elevated homocysteine levels as possibly contributing to lowered sperm count in males.

What are normal levels?

A healthy homocysteine reading or 'H' score is ideally less than 7 (reference range 0-15). However, a reading of 11 or 12 would still be considered normal (based on the current reference range) when in fact, a reading of 9 or above increases your chance of heart disease by two times. So, it makes sense to try to achieve a reading below 7 for optimal health.

If your levels of homocysteine are higher than 7, it is important to consult a practitioner who has experience with nutritional supplementation and its effects on the body.

Nutritional medicine to control homocysteine levels

B vitamins, in particular folic acid (or active folate if you have a gene mutation), vitamin B6 and vitamin B12 supplements work together to maintain healthy homocysteine levels.

Fortunately, the right nutritional supplements should make a difference in your homocysteine levels in just two months.

One study showed a two-fold increase of follicular fluid folate corresponded with a 3.3 times higher chance of achieving pregnancy in IVF.

Boxmeer JC et.al IVF outcomes are associated with biomarkers of the homocysteine pathway in monofollicular fluid. Hum. Reprod. 2009 May; 24(5):1059-66.

A daily supplement programme for lowering high homocysteine may include:

- Vitamin B6 100mg
- Vitamin B12 100mcg
- Folic acid 800mcg (or active folate 1mg).

The amounts you need will depend on your current homocysteine level, and your associated risk factors.

Reducing alcohol and caffeine, not smoking, avoiding salt, eating plenty of fruit and vegetables, and having less meat, more fish and vegetarian proteins such as beans and lentils have all been shown to lower homocysteine levels too.

Notes

MTHFR GENE MUTATION

A thorough discussion of MTHFR gene mutations would be as long as this book. My goal is to give you a basic understanding as it relates to fertility and pregnancy.

What is MTHFR?

MTHFR (5,10-methylenetetrahydrofolate reductase) is a gene found on a specific chromosome within every cell in every person. The MTHFR gene produces an enzyme responsible for a multi-step process that converts the amino acid homocysteine to another amino acid, methionine. The body uses methionine to make proteins and other important compounds.

What is a MTHFR mutation?

An abnormal change in gene structure, called a mutation, of the MTHFR gene can disrupt the MTHFR enzyme's normal function of breaking down homocysteine.

MTHFR mutations are common. Those of us with a MTHFR gene mutation have a highly reduced ability to convert folic acid or even folate into a usable form. Research estimates that as much as half of the population may have an MTHFR gene mutation, though there are many variations of the mutation, depending on how the gene was passed down from the parents. The C677T gene variant is the most widely researched, with the A1298 less so.

How does MTHFR affect fertility and pregnancy?

If the MTHFR gene is malfunctioning, homocysteine can build up and cause problems in the cardiovascular system and affect fertility and pregnancy.

Left undiagnosed, this gene mutation may lead to a variety of issues including difficulties conceiving, unexplained infertility, recurrent miscarriages and pre-eclampsia in pregnancy.

In addition, people with MTHFR gene defect may have lower levels of S-adenosylmethionine (SAMe), which has been shown to increase the likelihood of depression and postpartum depression. SAMe also plays an important role in immune system function, growth, repair and maintenance of cells, and is anti-inflammatory. All of these are critical in reproductive function and proper development of a baby in pregnancy.

Some MTHFR mutations are more serious than others as far as their ability to cause problems during pregnancy. Specifically, women who have multiple miscarriages are more likely to have a MTHFR gene mutation. Women who have the homozygous form of the MTHFR gene mutation (both of her alleles having the mutation) are at a more than two-fold increased risk for miscarriage.

The association of MTHFR and recurrent miscarriage is still being researched. Some researchers feel that the mutations can cause blood clots between the developing placenta and uterine wall, thus preventing transport of vital nutrients to the developing foetus. This usually occurs early in pregnancy when the embryo or foetus is most vulnerable.

It is unlikely that we will work out exactly how the MTHFR gene mutation affects pregnancy loss in the near future. For now, there is no set 'standard of care' protocol for dealing with recurrent miscarriage in the presence of a MTHFR mutation.

Testing for MTHFR gene mutation

If you have had failed IVF cycles, experienced recurrent miscarriages or any of the other pregnancy-related issues mentioned previously, ask your doctor or naturopath to arrange a MTHFR genetic test.

Saliva or blood samples may be obtained for testing. This should be carried out before you embark on another IVF cycle.

Results matter – heterozygous or homozygous?

The gene mutations can be 'heterozygous', meaning they occur only on one strand or 'allele' of the chromosome (have one copy), or they can be 'homozygous', occurring on both alleles (have two copies).

Those with homozygous MTHFR C677T are often advised to take their folate requirements more seriously. Homozygous individuals need to avoid synthetic folic acid; rather, they require a bioactive methylfolate in a supplement form.

What you can do if you test positive for MTHFR

You may feel overwhelmed if you are diagnosed with a genetic defect. However, this defect is quite common and fortunately there are steps you can take to counteract such a gene mutation:

- Eat a diet rich in naturally occurring folate, preferably from organic sources such as uncooked dark leafy green vegetables, asparagus, lentils, beans, papaya, grapefruit, walnuts and avocado.*
- Avoid processed foods that are fortified with synthetic folic acid (homozygous) or strictly limit them (heterozygous).
- Avoid both black and green tea as they can inhibit folate absorption.
- Avoid antacids as these also inhibit absorption of folate.
- Avoid supplementing with synthetic folic acid; choose a prenatal multivitamin that contains preferably methylated folate (homozygous) or folinic acid (heterozygous).
- If you are homozygous for the gene, you may need to take additional folate such as L-5-Methyltetrahydrofolate)

800mcg - 1mg per day (be guided by your doctor or naturopath).

- Continue to take 5-MTHFR throughout your pregnancy, not just the first trimester.
- Make sure all the B vitamins you supplement provide the methylated/bioactive form. For vitamin B6, this would be Pyridoxal 5-Phosphate or P5P; for Vitamin B12 this is methylcobalamin.
- Vegans may also require methylcobalamin and choline.

Caveat: Eating a folate–rich diet is not always the answer to ensuring adequate blood levels of folate if you have a MTHFR gene mutation.

'I eat so much green leafy veg and yet my folate levels are low'

Consider this scenario. You may be eating loads of kale and drinking green smoothies, yet you are still low in B12 and folate. Why?

We can saturate our cells with wholefood sources of folate and yet we may be worse off because it still needs to be broken down into methylated folate to be absorbed. In this situation, take folate in a bioactive supplement form, ideally in conjunction with a bioactive B complex to help extract more folate for the body to use.

For more information on MTHFR, refer to mthfr.net

Genes are never a marker of our destiny; rather, they are a marker of susceptibility.

IMMUNE ISSUES

Researchers now believe women who suffer recurrent miscarriages or IVF failures could have an immune system that is too healthy, consistently rejecting any invading cells, including the dad-to-be genes.

In fact, 50 per cent of miscarriages with no known male cause are due to immune dysfunction.

When immune issues are involved in miscarriage, the chances of a woman having a successful pregnancy without treatment:

- After three miscarriages is 30 per cent
- After four miscarriages is 25 per cent
- After five miscarriages is 5 per cent.

It is important you seek expert help and request a referral to see a reproductive immunologist, especially for older women.

One of my patients had tried several IVF cycles at various clinics in the UK, when finally, the couple had success at an IVF clinic in Athens, Greece. She was diagnosed with an immune system problem whereby her body was producing too many 'natural killer' cells (NK cells) that protect against invasion and infection. She was then referred to a reproductive immunologist who successfully controlled the dysfunction within her immune system. Nine months later she gave birth to a beautiful IVF-conceived baby girl.

By weakening a woman's immune system at the time of conception, doctors say they can significantly improve the chances of pregnancy. They may prescribe blood-thinning medicines and steroids for repeated miscarriages and IVF failures where immune issues such as elevated NK cells are detected.

In relation to NK cells issues, up to 25 per cent of women who have repeated miscarriage or IVF failure have high levels of NK cells. These can be detected through a blood test. A doctor may then prescribe a low dose of steroid (prednisolone) and blood-thinning medicine (clexane) to help suppress the NK cells, leading to a better chance of conception. Prescribed correctly, these medications are safe, and they work. Generally, women take the medication from the beginning of their cycle, until the third month of their pregnancy.

Naturopathic support for immune issues

Although naturopaths can't change the autoimmune diagnosis, we can recommend changes that lower the triggers for an autoimmune event.

Your naturopath may recommend:

- A low allergenic diet that avoids gluten, dairy and/or soy - in the case of thyroid antibodies, I always advise (insist!) my patients avoid gluten
- Antioxidant-rich foods and superfoods
- Low-acid foods to reduce inflammation
- Supplements to help modulate the immune system and dampen down the production of auto antibodies and reduce allergic response, such as vitamins C and D, zinc and probiotics
- Herbal medicines that support and treat autoimmune conditions including:
    - Echinacea – a powerful immune balancing, immune enhancing and anti-inflammatory herb. It is safe to use in autoimmune conditions. The preferred species is Echinacea angustifolia.
    - Hemidesmus – provides a unique natural immune depressant effect that dampens autoimmune antibody production.
    - Licorice and Rehmannia – both of these down regulate auto-immune acting cells – think of them as nature's natural prednisolone.

- Other herbs that also may be recommended include Albizia, Baical Skullcap, Ginkgo, Feverfew, Coleus and Withania.

N.B. Do not self-prescribe or take any of the above herbs unless they are recommended by a registered, experienced naturopath or medical herbalist who has a thorough knowledge of IVF procedures.

Notes

CLOTTING DISORDERS

Clotting disorders are a group of genetic disorders of the blood clotting pathways, leading to abnormal clot formation. These disorders can cause complications leading to miscarriage, stillborn births, pre-eclampsia (toxaemia of pregnancy), elevated liver enzymes and a low platelet count.

There are a number of gene mutations that lead to inherited thrombophilias:

- Factor V Leiden - most common type, occurring in approximately10 per cent of the Caucasian population. This is a major cause of blood clots associated with the oral contraceptive pill
- Prothrombin (factor II) – occurs in approximately 7 per cent of women who experience a foetal loss due to a clotting disorder
- MTHFR gene mutation - women who have the homozygous form of this gene mutation (both alleles having the mutation) have more than a two-fold increased risk of miscarriage (See Section 3, MTHFR Gene Mutations).

Pharmaceutical treatment for thrombophilias

Your doctor may prescribe aspirin or clexane (enoxaparin sodium) for up to 18 or even 24 weeks prior to starting an IVF cycle.

Fermented food as medicine

The traditional Japanese food Natto, containing an enzyme called nattokinase, has been used safely for more than 1,000 years to help dissolve blood clots.

Natto is produced by adding the bacteria '*Bacillus subtillis* to boiled soybeans. The resulting nattokinase enzyme is produced when the bacteria acts on the soybeans. While other soy foods contain enzymes, it is only the natto preparation that contains the nattokinase enzyme. If you can handle the taste and texture(!), this is a great adjunct to your IVF diet and supplement plan.

Other naturopathic adjunctive treatment includes:

- Fish oils capsules – up to 6000mg per day
- Supplemental nattokinase - 200-400mg per day (very expensive!)
- Herbal medicine such as Hemidesmus, Ginkgo biloba, Ginger and Turmeric
- Methylated folate (in cases of MTHFR gene mutation)
- Vitamin C with bioflavanoids – 2-3g per day
- Enteric-coated high potency garlic – 2-3 tablets per day
- Coenzyme Q10 – 150-300mg per day
- Vitamin E: up to 2000 IU per day.

LUTEAL PHASE DEFECTS

Luteal Phase Defect (LPD) occurs when the uterine lining (endometrium) is inadequately prepared and is too thin. This can contribute to infertility, implantation failure and early miscarriage.

Normally, the uterine lining grows 1 to 2mm every other day in response to oestrogen. After ovulation, a lining of between 8 and 13mm is considered normal. If the lining doesn't develop to this thickness, it is harder for an embryo to implant.

If the uterine lining doesn't develop properly, it may be because both oestrogen and progesterone production is low; the secretion of progesterone by the ovary is below normal; or because the endometrium isn't responding to the normal stimulation by progesterone.

Other reasons may include infection, scarring from dilation and curettages, poor uterine blood supply and sometimes endometrial antibodies.

Your doctor or specialist may assess this via blood tests and by two biopsies (because sporadic cycles with luteal phase defect can occur in any woman).

Your IVF specialist will usually offer the following treatment:

- Clomiphene citrate (oral) or FSH injections to stimulate follicular growth
- Supplemental hCG injections to improve secretion of progesterone post-embryo transfer
- Additional progesterone after egg retrieval surgery usually prescribed as vaginal suppositories or gel, or orally and through injections.

Naturopathic support

Certain foods such as phytoestrogens may assist in building up a healthy endometrium. The term 'phytoestrogen' means a plant-derived compound able to behave like an oestrogen and bind to the cell receptor to provide a weak oestrogenic effect where levels are low.

Examples of phytoestrogens include fermented soy products, alfalfa sprouts, red clover sprouts, lentils, kidney beans, split peas, green beans, fennel, fenugreek and other grains and seeds.

The use of supplements such as Vitamin B6 has demonstrated improvements in LPD.

During the preconception months, prior to the commencement of IVF medications, herbal medicine may be prescribed to support and balance both the follicular phase and the luteal phase of the cycle to assist in regulating the length of the luteal phase. Herbs may include Tribulus (has been shown to assist in restoring regular ovulation when prescribed on day 5 to day 14 of the menstrual cycle[18]) Chaste tree, Peony and Licorice, among others.

My 'trifecta' to assist with LPD prior to an IVF cycle is vitamin B6, Peony and Licorice prescribed from day 15 until the onset of menstruation. Vitamin B6 may be taken after egg retrieval, alongside progesterone prescribed by your doctor for LPD.

In addition, I advise patients to try the 'Seeding Protocol'...

[18] Zarkova S. Tribestan: Experimental and Clinical Investigations. Chemical Pharmaceutical Research Institute, Sofia, Bulgaria.

The Seeding Protocol – seed cycling

Seed cycling is a treatment to normalise menstrual cycles that I have used clinically with astounding success. The treatment helps restore consistency to irregular menstrual cycles where no obvious organic cause has been elicited or appears absent.

The seeding supports normal hormonal production. The flaxseeds and pumpkin seeds support the oestrogenic (follicular) phase, while the sesame and sunflower seeds support the progesterone (luteal) phase. Much of this work comes from Dr Christiane Northup's book, 'Women's Bodies, Women's Wisdom (Revised Edition): Creating Physical and Emotional Health and Healing'.

I have done this with many women, regardless of the cause of menstrual irregularities, and seen its efficacy. It usually takes three cycles for full effect.

How it works

Regardless of your cycle, on day 1 of the next New Moon through to day 15, have 1 tablespoon daily of organic ground flaxseeds and 1 tablespoon of ground pumpkin seeds. On days 16-28, have 1 tablespoon of ground sunflower seeds and 1 tablespoon of sesame seeds.

I suggest the following if you don't want to do the seeds.

- Days 1-15: take a quality, pure fish oil (total 1500-2000mg of EPA/DHA daily) three capsules daily, divided dose – morning and night)
- Days 16-28: take two 500mg capsules of Gamma-linolenic acid (GLA) daily, divided dose.

Notes

Section 4

Dietary Requirements for Each Phase of IVF

Following the guidelines of an IVF diet is not dissimilar to the preconception diet guidelines outlined in this book.

If you have already been following a healthy preconception diet, you would have been laying the groundwork for a specific IVF diet.

The emphasis once again is on a Mediterranean wholefoods diet, including plenty of high-quality protein, fruit, vegetables and healthy fats. Foods rich in healthy fats such as avocados, nuts and seeds, free-range organic eggs and coconut oil provide necessary nutrition for healthy hormone balance. Fruit and vegetables alongside superfoods provide important antioxidant support to protect the egg and sperm's journey from beginning to conception.

What's more, going gluten-free is another step to consider in your IVF journey. Your naturopath may advise if this is a consideration for you. I certainly suggest eating gluten-free foods to my patients if they exhibit signs and symptoms that suggest a gluten intolerance e.g. infertility.

As Hippocrates said

'Let food be thy medicine'

GOING GLUTEN FREE

If you follow nutrition and fertility news, you may have read that gluten sensitivity and/or coeliac disease (a disease of the small intestine caused by gluten allergy) may be linked to infertility and irregularities with the menstrual cycle. In fact, screening for coeliac disease and/or gluten intolerance should be a priority in infertile women and couples.

What is gluten?

Gluten is a protein found in barley, oats, rye and wheat. Gluten intolerance or sensitivity is when a person reacts to gluten. This reaction may be severe, such as the symptoms of coeliac disease, or more subtle such as unexplained weight gain, low energy, poor concentration and hormone imbalances.

Many people who are sensitive to gluten containing grains may not necessarily have an autoimmune reaction to gluten, making testing not always conclusive.

Hormone and reproductive problems associated with gluten sensitivity

Research studies have shown that women with gluten sensitivity are more likely to experience:

- Polycystic Ovarian Syndrome (PCOS)
- Pelvic Inflammatory Disorders (PID)
- Endometriosis
- Hypothyroidism, Hashimoto's and Graves's disease
- Amenorrhoea and Hypothalamic amenorrhoea
- Delays in menstruation
- Infertility (in men, infertility is reflected in low sperm count and low motility)
- Miscarriage
- Gynaecological and obstetric complications
- Low birth weight.

In clinical practice, I find up to 80 per cent of women with infertility due to PCOS test positive to gluten sensitivity. When these women remove gluten from their diets, they often see marked improvements in their PCOS symptoms, not to mention weight loss, improved cholesterol levels and thyroid health, and often, pregnancy!

Other symptoms and conditions that may be associated with a gluten intolerance include:

- Digestive upset – bloating, diarrhoea, and even constipation (most people I treat who have chronic constipation since childhood have a gluten intolerance)
- Fatigue or brain fog after eating meals containing wheat/gluten
- Autoimmune disease
- Neurological symptoms – dizziness, feeling off balance
- Migraines
- Chronic fatigue and fibromyalgia
- Swelling in hands, feet and legs
- Mood disorders – anxiety, depression and mood swings
- Painful joints and muscle stiffness.

Testing for gluten intolerance

Depending on where you are in the world, gluten sensitivity testing can be expensive and may not be covered by your private health insurance fund.

In preparation for a blood test, it is important that you consume gluten in some form (wheat, barley, rye, oats) at the time of the test (for at least six weeks). The following tests may be performed:

- HLA tissue typing for coeliac disease (genetic testing): HLA - DQ2 and DQ8. This test needs to be conducted first. If the results are positive, then the following tests will be required.

- Anti-Tissue Transglutaminase IgA antibodies and anti-endomysial antibodies (EMA), and/or
- Gluten withdrawal/challenge dietary test.

A gluten withdrawal/challenge test requires you to follow a strict gluten-free diet for a month. Record what you eat and any changes you may feel using a food diary. Then prepare for the challenge by eating gluten containing grains for a couple of days and note down any reactions - physical, mental and emotional. If you notice reactions and feel worse then you may well be gluten intolerant or have a gluten sensitivity.

Should you try a gluten-free diet?

I am seeing a significant rise in gluten intolerance/sensitivity in my clinic – both from positive tests (for coeliac markers or gluten intolerance), and in those patients who test negative but have many of the symptoms and simply feel much healthier on a gluten-free diet.

You may be pleasantly surprised by how easy and enjoyable a gluten-free diet can be, and how good you can feel, often in unexpected ways.

Benefits of gluten-free eating

The most common health benefits experienced from following a gluten-free diet include:

- Weight loss
- Increased energy
- Improved concentration
- Resolution of abdominal bloating and wind
- Resolution of constipation, diarrhoea and Irritable Bowel Syndrome (IBS)
- Improved mood
- Simply feeling better than usual!

Some dramatic hormone benefits may (hopefully!) include:

- Pregnancy
- Recovery from PCOS
- Recovery from PID
- Recovery from thyroid diseases such as Hashimoto's and Graves disease.

Gluten-free eating: all or nothing

If you are contemplating going gluten-free, it is 'all or nothing'. You need to remove every shred of gluten from your diet for your body to experience life without gluten continually passing through your gut.

One caveat here is that not all gluten-free foods are healthy or fertility promoting; many are made from white rice flour, refined corn starch, salt and sugar.

The goal of your gluten-free diet should be to restore hormone balance, lose weight and nourish your fertility, not simply replace gluten with processed, pre-packaged and sugary gluten-free foods, of which there are many.

A gluten-free diet is a great opportunity to have less flour-based foods and increase your intake of fruits, vegetables, wholegrains, beans and good quality proteins.

The grains that you need to avoid are wheat (bulgar, semolina, cous cous, seitan), spelt, triticale, kamut, rye and barley. Oats contain a gluten-like property called Avenin (i.e. oat gluten), which only one in 10,000 Westerners may have an intolerance to.

Traditionally, most oats are grown as a rotational crop in wheat, barley, triticale and rye fields. This can cross-contaminate the oat with such grains (this may also happen in processing). So it is important to obtain oats grown strictly in fields with no other cereal crop to avoid cross-contamination.

Glutinous grains sneak into many foods and beverages such as beer, malt vinegar, malt flavouring, soy sauce (you can buy a gluten-free kind or substitute with tamari), communion wafers, stock cubes, gravy and sauce mixes.

The message here: READ YOUR LABELS!

Refer to *The IVF Diet Cookbook* for gluten-free meal suggestions.

Notes

FOOD GROUPS

Learning about nutrition - including the main food groups - will give you a greater understanding of what a balanced diet means and make it easier for you to follow the IVF diet outlined in this book. Learning more about nutrition will also help you make good food choices to lose extra weight if this is a concern for you.

Carbohydrates

Carbohydrates provide energy, essential vitamins and minerals, and valuable fibre which act like a 'broom' to keep your digestive tract healthy and clean. Your body needs good quality carbohydrates for energy. Eating the right type (quality) and the right amount (quantity) can make all the difference between you having a lean healthy body or carrying extra weight.

Different carbohydrates have different effects on your body. The Glycemic Index (GI) is a numerical rating that compares the effect of different carbohydrates on your blood sugar levels.

Choosing foods with a low GI ranking is critical for women who are carrying extra weight or have PCOS as these foods prevent blood sugar levels from spiking suddenly, thereby reducing the insulin response. This can reduce excessive hormone release from the ovaries and allow the body to burn more fat. Eating low GI foods can also keep your energy levels stable for longer and reduce sweet cravings.

Low GI foods

Refined carbohydrates such as doughnuts, bagels, white bread, biscuits and sweets are off the menu! Instead, choose complex carbohydrates such as fruit, vegetables and low GI gluten-free wholegrains, which are all high in fibre.

Here are a few tips:

- Eat more low GI foods such as gluten-free breads (see my quinoa bread recipe in the *IVF cookbook*), oats, apples, basmati rice and sweet potato.
- Be careful when choosing your grains. Most grains are high in nutrients and have a low GI value but not all. Food that is high in amylopectin (a type of enzyme) such as wheat, corn and most types of rice are broken down rapidly and classified as high GI foods. Even brown rice (nutrient-rich but high GI) should be eaten in moderation if you need to lose weight. Examples of low GI grains are buckwheat, kamult, basmati rice, rye, spelt (not these two if you are gluten-free) and quinoa (which is technically a seed).
- If you need to lose weight, watch your quantities of carbs and only have 1/3 cup cooked rice/pasta, 15g cereal, ½ cup cooked oats or one slice of bread per serve/meal.

Low GL foods

The Glycemic Load (GL) index is based on the GI index, and considers the typical serving size of each type of food and the amount of carbohydrates in that serving. These values are more precise in terms of the amount of food you would normally be expected to eat. Foods with high GL values will raise your blood sugar faster than those with low GL values. Examples of low GL foods include most high-fibre fruit and vegetables, legumes such as kidney beans, chick peas, pinto beans and lentils.

Fibre

A fibre-rich diet is important, as fibre helps to maintain healthy digestive function, keep your bowel movements regular, aid proper excretion of excess hormones and slow the absorption of sugar into the bloodstream.

Fibre-rich foods include gluten-free wholegrains, fruit, vegetables, nuts and seeds (including hormone-balancing flaxseeds), and legumes.

> An easy way to increase your fibre intake is with psyllium husks. These are light and fluffy flakes that you can sprinkle on cereal or add to smoothies. They absorb a lot of water when passing through the digestive tract, expanding the contents of the gut, which press against the intestinal wall to stimulate peristalsis (the movement of food through the digestive tract, enhancing bowel regularity).
>
> **N.B.** When increasing fibre intake, it is important to also increase water intake, otherwise you may experience stomach discomfort. Aim for six to eight glasses of water each day.

Vegetables

Vegetables are abundant in nutrients and fibre, and low in fat and calories. Cruciferous vegetables, such as broccoli, cabbage, brussels sprouts, bok choy and cauliflower contain Diindolylmethane (DIM), a phytochemical that improves oestrogen metabolism. It helps to detoxify excess oestrogen and convert it to a more beneficial form. To produce this chemical, the vegetables must be chopped and cooked or fermented.

Raw cruciferous vegetables contain thyroid inhibitors known as goitrogens. These may reduce thyroid function so if you have an underactive thyroid you should lightly steam or cook these vegetables for six to seven minutes to break down the goitrogens. Fermenting also deactivates goitrogenic activity e.g. eat sauerkraut instead of raw cabbage.

N.B: Be guided by your healthcare practitioner in regards to fermented foods if you have elevated histamine levels as they may not be advisable.

From a weight loss point of view, have maximum two cups of vegetables per serve. Limit the higher-starch vegetables such as corn, peas, sweet potato (kumura) and potato to one cup maximum twice per week.

Fruits

Fruits are nutrient-rich and high in fibre, assisting with bowel regularity. The sugar in fruit is called fructose and when this is naturally occurring with fibre, and in moderation, is a good choice to help curtail sugar cravings.

If you need to lose weight, choose your fruits carefully as the ratio of glucose to fructose determines which fruits have a higher GI. For example, grapes (especially black grapes) are high in glucose, compared to fructose; whereas apples are higher in fructose than glucose. Stone fruits, melons and berries have lower GI values. Avoid fruit juices, stewed fruit and dried fruit. By consuming fruit in a different form, the fibre content is distorted, and the sugar content is usually tripled, contributing to weight gain.

Beware of sugar!

Sugar is bad news! Sugar will not only worsen insulin resistance and contribute to weight gain but will also accelerate the inflammatory response. Sugar overloads the control mechanisms in your body.

Sugars have many names:

Glucose	Galactose	Xylitol	Malt/malt extract
Dextrose	Fructose	Sorbitol	Corn starch
Sucrose	Mannose	Mannitol	Modified carbohydrate
Maltose	Lactose	Raw sugar	Brown sugar
Golden syrup	Honey	White sugar	Rice syrup

Here are a few tips:

- Avoid foods with added sugar, including artificial sweeteners, which lead to greater carbohydrate cravings and weaker insulin resistance.

- Read all labels for sugar and the type of sugar used. Limit refined sugar as much as possible and enjoy fructose in the way Mother Nature intended - by eating two to three serves of fruit daily.

Nutritional panels on packaged goods can be confusing. Here's a quick way to tell if you're consuming too much sugar, fat or salt: instead of looking at the 'per serve' column, look at the 'per 100g' or 'per 100ml' column. This will give you a much better insight as serving sizes differ widely.

For example, saturated fat falls into an acceptable range at 0-2g per 100g, or 0-0.9g per 100ml, but is not acceptable at 15g or more per 100g or 7g or more per 100ml. For sugar, a 'good' range is 0-6g per 100g or 0-3g per 100ml; 'bad' would be over 9g per 100g or 5g per 100ml. With salt, a 'good' level would be 0-130mg per 100g or 0-130mg for 100ml; a 'bad' one would be 350mg per 100g or 350mg per 100ml.

A note on fructose

Fructose is found in fruit and foods such as corn syrup, which is added to soft drinks and processed foods including some yoghurts and fruit spreads. It is fine to consume small amounts of fructose combined with fibre i.e. in whole fruit. However, we are doing the opposite by consuming large amounts of fructose with negligible fibre. Fructose without the fibre can damage our liver cells, in turn causing high blood pressure and increasing fats in the blood. The other issue is that our body will metabolise more fructose than is needed. This can result in increased fat storage (hence weight gain) and the production of free radicals (which may damage cells in the heart and liver).

Protein

Protein is necessary to build muscle, fight disease, protect the skin, make hormones and for enzymes that keep our cells working. It is also essential for follicle growth and egg quality.

The building blocks of proteins, called amino acids, are essential for life. Nine of the 20 amino acids cannot be made by the body, so must be supplied by food. If there is inadequate protein intake then new cells cannot be made, nor can the enzymes or hormones be made that enable these cells to operate.

Complete and incomplete proteins

Some proteins are 'complete', others are 'incomplete', and you need them both.

'Complete' protein (containing the nine essential amino acids your body needs) is found mainly in meat, fish, chicken, eggs, protein powders, quinoa and superfoods such as spirulina.

Complementary proteins are incomplete proteins as they may lack some of the essential amino acids. These include fruits, vegetables, grains, seeds, nuts and beans. If you follow a vegetarian-based diet, it is important to eat a wide variety of plant-based protein at every meal to make sure you get the full spectrum of essential amino acids.

Protein should be part of every meal, including snacks. Preferred protein foods include fish and seafood (not prawns), lean organic chicken, grass-fed beef and lamb, lentils, legumes, nuts, seeds, quinoa, organic cheese and yoghurt (if dairy tolerant), coconut yoghurt, organic eggs, superfoods and protein powders such as whey protein isolate, golden pea/hemp/sprouted rice protein.

From a weight loss point of view, eating protein with each meal stabilises your blood sugar levels, provide a steady supply of energy and a feeling of fullness and satisfaction for hours.

Protein: Carbohydrate ratio to lose excess weight

The rate of protein to carbohydrate in a meal is important, especially regarding weight loss. An easy ratio to implement, which will give approximately the right proportions, is to balance each meal, snack or plate with 1:1 volume. Then assess the carbohydrate portion for overall GL value.

So, no more plates of pasta or rice with sauce! These foods should be seen as an accompaniment to, rather than the basis of a meal.

Here are a few more tips:

- The smaller the animal and the fewer legs it has, the less saturated fat it contains.

- Include **legumes** and pulses in your diet, as both are low GL, low in fat and high in dietary fibre (good for bowel regularity). Soak dry legumes overnight and discard soaking water.

- Eat **nuts** and **seeds** as they contain good fats. However, they can turn rancid very quickly if not stored in the fridge (or even frozen if you do not intend to eat them within two weeks). Stale nuts can cause a damaging free radical cascade. Nuts that taste stale or bitter should be discarded. Avoid roasted and salted varieties. You can also soak nuts and seeds to deactivate the phytates to assist digestion. Soaking time will vary depending on the nut or seed e.g. soak almonds overnight, soak cashews just six hours (otherwise they go soggy.)

- Choose cold water **fish** high in **essential fatty acids** such as herring, salmon, mackerel, mullet and sardines. Avoid fish with higher contamination levels (especially mercury) such as swordfish, tuna, and shark (flake). Check which fish have lower contamination levels in your area.

- Avoid or minimise your dairy intake, as all dairy foods will increase saturated fat. Low-fat dairy foods are highly processed and may contain added sugar, vegetable oils, artificial sweeteners or food additives. If you drink milk, look for goat's and sheep's milk and milk products, which are more easily digested than cow's milk (except yoghurt, which is pre-digested, and A2 milk, which does not contain the A1 protein, often responsible for allergies). If you are using butter, make sure it is organic.

- Choose milk alternatives such as rice, oat, quinoa, hemp, almond or coconut milk.

A note on soy

Some research has suggested soy is detrimental to fertility. However, in many cultures, soy is a staple food and their level of infertility is no higher than our own. In a normal mixed diet, including a small amount of pre-soaked or fermented soy three to four times a week is helpful, especially for vegetarians and vegans to provide some protein, calcium and iron. Ensure it is organic and GM-free. Natto is to be considered, especially if thrombophilia is an issue.

However, unfermented soy (soy milk, soy yoghurt, soy cheese and tofu) should be avoided, as it contains phytates and enzyme inhibitors, which will prevent protein and mineral absorption. This form also dampens thyroid activity. Also watch for added soy in baked products such as soy lecithin, soy flour and soy oil. If you can't help but have a square of chocolate every now and then, cacao butter in chocolate is a better choice than soy lecithin.

Fats and oils

Healthy fats

In the past, fats were blamed for everything from weight gain to heart disease and cancer. We now know that there are good fats and bad fats. The good fats are mono- and poly-unsaturated fats, as well as essential fatty acids (EFAs).

The Mediterranean diet emphasises healthy fats as part of a wholefood diet.

The best fats for hormone health are Omega 3 and Omega 6 EFAs. Omega 3 fats are abundant in deep sea oily fish like salmon, sardines and tuna, and in flaxseed (linseed) oil. Omega 6 EFAs are found in evening primrose oil and some vegetable oils. However, the problem is that while it is easy to consume Omega 6 EFAs, it is not as easy to consume Omega 3 EFAs as they are mostly in fish. The optimum ratio of Omega 3 to Omega 6 is three to one.

Healthy fats can be found in:

- *Omega 3*: sardines, anchovies, salmon, mackerel, mullet, flaxseed oil, egg yolk, nuts and vegetable oils
- *Omega 6:* evening primrose oil, GLA flaxseed, borage (containing gamma linolenic acid, GLA) and blackcurrant
- *Monounsaturated fats:* olives, avocado, nuts, sunflower oil
- *Coconut oil:* use only good quality virgin coconut oil, preferably organic. It should contain no fillers, added oils or other additives. It will be solid at room temperature. Many people have been told to avoid coconut oil because it contains a high amount of saturated fats; however, not all saturated fats are equal. Coconut oil is rich in beneficial saturated fats like lauric acid, which actually benefits the thyroid, heart, brain and gut.
- *Other sources:* organic butter, mayonnaise, olive, tahini, nuts.

Bad fats

'Bad' fats (saturated, damaged and trans fats) need to be avoided as much as possible as they compete with EFAs for uptake, thereby affecting hormone balance.

Margarine should be avoided. It is a highly processed food that contains trans fats, a source of free radicals that can cripple or kill cells. Beware of enticing names such as 'olive oil spread', which sound healthy but are quite the opposite.

Other foods to avoid include organ meats, fat in red meat, pastries and commercially baked cookies, doughnuts and muffins, and processed food.

Oils for cooking

One would think any oil suffices for cooking. This is NOT the case. Non-processed and organic saturated fats (the kind that are solid or semi-solid at room temperature) are typically the best for cooking at high temperatures, as they will not go rancid nor oxidise.

What does this mean? When oil goes rancid or oxidises, it produces free radicals. Free radicals cause premature ageing and diseases.

So, when cooking at high temperatures or with a high flame you should use a good quality saturated oil or fat that will remain stable when being heated and not produce any free radicals. Such fats are coconut oil, sesame oil, butter (preferably organic butter from grass-fed cows) or ghee.

When using a low flame, or baking food in the oven, monounsaturated cold-pressed extra virgin olive oil is a good choice. Olive oil will go rancid and create free radicals at high temperatures (or with a high flame).

Rice bran oil is a little more stable than grapeseed oil and can be used for very low-heat applications, but rice bran oil still has a high polyunsaturated content so it's best to store it in the fridge and use in moderate amounts.

A good general rule of thumb: if you're cooking with more than a medium flame on the stove-top, don't use olive oil or rice bran oil. Use coconut, butter or ghee instead (depending on what you are cooking).

So, what is the best oil to cook with?

The best oil to cook with is coconut oil. Coconut oil is stable when cooking at higher temperatures and it has incredible health benefits including weight loss, improved thyroid function and enhanced immune function. It also helps keep the skin looking young and healthy. When purchasing coconut oil, it is important to use organic coconut oil. You will find coconut oil/butter in health food stores.

If you find the smell of coconut overwhelming, 'odourless' coconut oils are available.

Here is a list so you know what to cook with and when:

- Pan-fried eggs: only use coconut oil, organic butter or ghee
- Grilled/pan-fried chicken: only use coconut oil, organic butter or ghee
- Baked chicken: use olive oil, not extra virgin (when baking or using a low flame on the stove-top)
- Grilled/pan-fried fish: only use coconut oil, organic butter or ghee
- Grilled/BBQ/pan-fried meat: only use coconut oil, organic butter or ghee. Don't use olive oil to cook meat.

H_2O: The good drop

Water is vital for life. It is needed to transport nutrients, rid the body of waste products and maintain regular bowel movements. You can feel very bloated during the follicular phase of an IVF cycle (priming of the follicles with FSH injections) as time goes on, especially just prior to egg retrieval surgery. It is also important to keep well hydrated after surgery and embryo transfer, so you don't get constipated. Depending on the filtration unit, filtering water can remove unwanted chlorine and fluoride.

You should aim to:

- Drink two litres of filtered water a day (including herbal decaffeinated teas) but avoid drinking with meals as this dilutes digestive enzymes and reduces the absorption of important nutrients.
- Add one litre of water per hour of exercise. It is a good idea to hydrate well before, during and after your workout to replenish lost fluid stores.

IVF DIET GUIDELINES

When embarking on an IVF cycle, optimal nutrition is essential. There is much research to suggest following a healthy, nutrient-rich diet will maximise a positive IVF outcome.

Eating well and with awareness is the key to optimising nutrition. Below are some tips to help you stay on track and consume the right foods.

Eating a Mediterranean Diet May Increase Chance of Pregnancy in Couples Undergoing IVF-ICSI Treatment

In a study involving 161 couples undergoing IVF/ICSI treatment, results indicate that eating a Mediterranean diet rich in vegetable oils, vegetables, fish, legumes and low intakes of snacks was positively associated with a 40 per cent increased chance of pregnancy.

'The preconception Mediterranean dietary pattern in couples undergoing in vitro fertilization/intracytoplasmic sperm injection treatment increases the chance of pregnancy', Vujkovic M, Steegers-Theunissen RP, et al, Fertil Steril, 2010 Feb 18.

Dietary guidelines when undergoing IVF

- Eat organic if possible, with emphasis on cruciferous vegetables.
- Ensure adequate fibre intake from fruit, vegetables and gluten-free wholegrains.
- Have quality protein with each meal, including protein-balancing snacks for morning and afternoon tea to stabilise blood sugar levels.
- Include good fats such as avocado, nuts, seeds, coconut oil and organic butter. This is what constitutes a Mediterranean-style diet.
- Drink two litres of filtered water daily. Decaffeinated herb teas can be included.

- Avoid refined carbohydrates. Cut out sugar (sweets, chocolate, cakes, biscuits, sugared soft drinks), jam, dried fruit, white flour products and fried food from your diet.
- Avoid or limit dairy. If you include dairy in your diet, organic is preferred.
- Avoid artificial sweeteners, preservatives and additives.
- Avoid alcohol and caffeine.
- Sit down for your meals. Eat slowly and with mindfulness.
- Eat regularly and don't skip meals. Allow a maximum of four hours between meals.
- Have breakfast every day to kick-start your metabolism for the day.
- When in doubt, leave it out.

My top 7 IVF foods

Below is a list of my top food choices to add to your IVF shopping trolley.

1. Organic fresh fruits and vegetables

It goes without saying that a healthy diet can create a healthy baby. To avoid pesticides and other food additives, eat organic fresh fruits and vegetables when possible. If you don't have access to them or can't afford them, be sure to wash with a dedicated vegetable wash or vinegar to remove pesticide residue. If you have a farmer's market near you, you can usually find very fresh produce in your area at a competitive price. You may even find some farmers in those markets entirely committed to organic produce.

Food for thought

A recent study on pregnancy diet and DNA has found that a mother's diet at the time of conception may affect the baby's genes. So, if you eat junk food before getting pregnant, you have a 50 per cent increased risk of giving birth prematurely.

genomebiology.com/2015/16/1/118

2. Apples

'An apple a day keeps the doctor away' as they say. Calcium D-Glucarate is a compound found in apples, grapefruit and cruciferous vegetables. This is converted to a compound that inhibits an enzyme that causes problems in the gut called beta-glucuronidase. High levels of this enzyme have been associated with oestrogen-dominant conditions such as fibroids, but also hormonally related cancers like breast, prostate and colon cancer. Other foods high in glucaric acid (a form of calcium D-glucarate) include bean sprouts, broccoli, brussels sprouts, cabbage and grapefruit.

N.B. Calcium D-glucarate can also be taken in a supplement form: three to four 500mg capsules twice a day.

3. Pineapple

This tropical fruit is rich in vitamin C, bioflavanoids and bromelain - an enzyme beneficial for combating inflammation and supporting the uterine lining. Chopped up and eaten on its own or as part of a fruit salad, this fruit lends itself to a delicious snack.

4. Healthy fats

Foods high in monounsaturated fats – including olive oil, sunflower oil, nuts, seeds and avocados – may boost IVF success rates for those who consume a good amount of these healthy fats. These foods, along with fruit, vegetables and quality protein such as fish, are what constitute a Mediterranean-style diet.

Research from the Harvard School of Public Health suggests eating avocados may triple live birth rates for couples undergoing IVF.[19]

Although such studies sound very promising, it is important not to place too much emphasis on one dietary recommendation as IVF success depends on a complex range of factors rather than just eating an avocado a day – if only!

[19] D.S. Colaci, M. Afeiche, A.J. Gaskins, D. Wright, T.L. Toth, R. Hauser, J.E. Chavarro et al.Dietary fat intake and in-vitro fertilization outcomes: saturated fat intake is associated with fewer metaphase oocytes Harvard School of Public Health, Boston MA, U.S.A. June 2012

5. Flaxseeds

Also, a source of healthy fats, these little seeds are rich in a vegetarian omega 3 EFAs, are anti-inflammatory and help with oestrogen clearance and balance. Add two tablespoons ground into smoothies or sprinkled over porridge or cereal daily.

6. Nuts

Almonds, Brazil nuts and macadamias are a great source of protein to eat on the go. Remember to store in the refrigerator to retain freshness.

7. Fermented foods

Live yoghurt, kefir (if dairy tolerant), sauerkraut, kimchi, miso and tempeh are examples of fermented foods which aid in the balance of beneficial gut bacteria, critical for a healthy immune system and digestive balance.

8. Superfoods

These are special natural foods that are packed full of goodness, including antioxidants and essential amino acids - nutrients we need but cannot make ourselves. Leafy green vegetables and dark-coloured berries are well known for their high nutrient content, and now foods like maca, mesquite, cacao and lucuma are gaining popularity. Such superfoods can be used as 'booster foods' to supplement a healthy, wholefood diet. Refer to Section 4, Superfoods for more details.

What to avoid

Alcohol

As noted in the preconception section, it is important to avoid alcohol prior to and during an IVF cycle and pregnancy. Excess alcohol may reduce your chances of conceiving by half.

Caffeine

Caffeine can also contribute to infertility and increase the chance of a miscarriage. Remember, it's not just coffee to avoid, but also black tea, green tea, energy drinks and, alas, chocolate.

Sugars

Too much sugar, especially white sugar, is not good for anyone. Artificial sweeteners should also be avoided. These can trigger inflammation, immune dysfunction, insulin resistance, tooth decay and of course contribute to weight gain and reproductive conditions such as PCOS.

Notes

DIETARY GUIDELINES FOR EACH STAGE OF THE IVF CYCLE

Here are some dietary guidelines for every stage of the IVF cycle.

The follicular development phase

During the follicular development phase, the main recommendation is to follow the IVF diet guidelines with an emphasis on quality protein and healthy fats.

Protein is essential for follicle growth and egg quality. In addition, foods rich in healthy fats such as avocados, nuts and seeds, free-range organic eggs, and coconut oil provide precursors for hormone synthesis and production.

Studies have proven women going through IVF produce more fertilised eggs at the blastocyst stage after eating more protein and less refined carbohydrates.

Another interesting study reviewed women who on previous IVF cycles had poorer blastocyst results. Two months before their next IVF cycle, the women were advised to increase their protein and reduce their refined carbohydrate intake. The result? Significantly higher blastocyst formation and higher pregnancy rates – again!

The egg retrieval phase

The main recommendation, apart from following the IVF diet guidelines, is to ensure bowel regularity is maintained and to prevent constipation.

Drink at least two litres of filtered water daily to aid elimination. Prune and pear juice are sometimes recommended if constipation becomes an issue. Pear juice may be preferred as it produces slightly less 'wind'!

It can be normal to feel a little sore and bloated after egg retrieval surgery, and you may not be in the mood to sit down to a proper dinner when you get home. A nice vegetable, lentil or chicken soup would be ideal.

Here is my 'Constipation Buster' recipe: a delicious way to fix an embarrassing problem.

Blend:

- 2 tsp flaxseeds, soaked overnight in ¼ cup boiling water
- 5 prunes, de-seeded (sulphur-free)
- ½ cup iced spring or filtered water
- ½ cup frozen banana, sliced
- ½ cup natural yoghurt (or coconut yoghurt if dairy-free)
- Optional addition of 1-2 tablespoons of protein powder

You can also replace banana (which makes it nice and creamy) with one kiwi fruit (including skin) and ½ cup ice.

Process all ingredients together, including any leftover flaxseed/linseed soaking water. Serve immediately. Makes one serve.

The embryo transfer phase

Continue with the IVF diet recommended guidelines. If you still feel slightly tender, continue to have lighter meals and soups and plenty of water at all times.

Additional dos and don'ts post-embryo transfer

- Don't lift heavy objects.
- Don't have sex.
- Don't exercise vigorously (gentle walking is fine).
- Do relax – meditate, listen to my audio '*Guided Meditation for IVF Success*', listen to music, read or watch a movie.

The luteal phase: post-embryo transfer

Are there foods you can eat to strengthen and build the uterine lining, which would in turn aid with implantation and ongoing pregnancy?

The short answer is that if you have followed a healthy preconception diet and recommended IVF guidelines, with an emphasis on healthy fats, quality protein, complex carbohydrates from gluten-free grains, fruit and vegetables, then you are in great shape for encouraging your lining to reach the thickness needed to support implantation — barring any underlying medical issue.

Your doctor will treat you for medical issues that cause problems with the uterine lining.

For more information, please refer to Section 3, Obstacles to Overcome: Luteal Phase Defects.

You can help increase your uterine lining with phytoestrogenic foods such as:

- Beans - split peas, millet, lentils, lima beans, chickpeas, black eyed peas, navy beans, red beans, mung bean sprouts.
- Grains and seeds - brown rice, oats, flaxseeds, sunflower seeds, pumpkin seeds.
- Vegetables - celery, beets, bok choy, broccoli, brussels sprouts, cauliflower, carrots, cucumbers, mushrooms, pumpkin, edible seaweeds, and tomatoes.
- Fruits - apples, cherries, pears, plums, prunes.
- Culinary herbs - ginger, oregano, sage, thyme, turmeric, cloves.

There are many ways to prepare and incorporate these foods in your diet but if you're looking for a quick phytoestrogen fix without a lot of preparation, try juicing, ideally with a Thermomix™, Vitamix™ or Nutribullet™ to ensure the fibre content remains.

Pineapple core may aid implantation

Eating pineapple, and specifically pineapple core, to aid implantation is a widespread theory and is also prescribed by natural and Chinese medicine practitioners. Although there is no clinical evidence as yet that pineapple helps implantation, it is worth trying (and reap the benefits of eating healthy fruit at the same time!)

Pineapple core contains an enzyme called bromelain that reduces inflammation and acts as a mild blood thinner, which is one reason why it may aid implantation.

Try eating one or two slices of pineapple each day (core intact – as the core contains the highest concentration of bromelain) from embryo transfer until pregnancy test day.

You won't be able to achieve the same results with canned pineapple, as the heating process for canning is destructive to bromelain. That means going out and finding a fresh, whole pineapple – sticking to organic whenever possible. The wedges can be stored in your refrigerator, and one pineapple should last you until implantation has occurred. Focus on enjoying your daily tropical fruit allowance, while envisioning a healthy embryo implanting safely into your uterus.

Foods to avoid

In the hopeful scenario that the embryo implants and you become pregnant, it is wise to avoid the following foods which may harbour Listeria or even Salmonella:

- Take-away cooked chickens
- Delicatessen meats and pates
- Pre-washed salads
- Soft cheeses
- Raw or undercooked meat, chicken and seafood including sushi and sashimi.

Continue to avoid caffeine and alcohol, and of course no smoking.

The frozen embryo (FET) cycle

Follow the recommended IVF diet guidelines pre- and post a frozen embryo transfer, including the dietary recommendations for the luteal phase.

Pregnancy

When you achieve a positive pregnancy test result, you will no doubt feel on top of the world. Once you have cried tears of joy, it is time to focus on healthy eating for both you and your developing baby. Dietary recommendations can be found in Section 9: When IVF Works.

Putting it all together

Try not to be overwhelmed by all this information. It will help to re-read this chapter and familiarise yourself with the information. You can do it!

It makes it easier if you think ahead, be organised and prepare menu plans and shopping lists. The following daily and weekly menu plan may be a useful guide. In addition, the companion book 'The IVF Diet Cookbook' provides inspirational and delicious recipes.

A typical day's menu

Upon rising	A glass of water with a squeeze/slice of lemon
Breakfast	1 selection each: protein, complex carbohydrate (from fruit/grain or both), good fat Herbal tea/chai almond latte
Morning tea	Green smoothie/protein shake Handful of nuts
Lunch	1 selection each: protein, salad/vegetables, grain (optional – especially if you need to lose weight), good fat
Afternoon tea	1 serve fruit and 30g nuts/ homemade protein ball Decaffeinated tea/herbal tea
Dinner	1 selection each: protein, salad/vegetables, good fat Dessert optional e.g. chia fruit pudding

Note: Drink two litres of filtered water a day but avoid drinking with meals as this dilutes digestive enzymes and reduces the absorption of important nutrients.

A Sample Weekly Menu

Meal	Monday	Tuesday	Wednesday	Thursday	Friday	Saturday	Sunday
Upon Rising	Hot water with lemon	Hot water with lemon	Hot water with lemon	Hot water with lemon	Hot water with lemon	Hot water with lemon	Hot water with lemon
Breakfast	Protein smoothie	Nut porridge	Poached eggs and avocado on quinoa toast	Paleo banana pancakes	Homemade gluten-free muesli	Buckwheat pancakes	Eggs Florentine and avocado
Snack	A piece of fruit and protein cookie	A piece of fruit and protein ball	A piece of fruit and protein bar	Protein smoothie or shake	A piece of fruit and handful of almonds	A piece of fruit and oat cakes with hummus	A piece of fruit and handful of nuts
Lunch	Butter bean and rosemary soup	Organic chicken salad	Hummus with vegan protein balls	Salad Nicoise	Veggie omelette	Salmon salad	Pumpkin and almond soup
Snack	A slice of Well Woman's Cake	Protein smoothie or shake	A piece of fruit and handful of almonds	A piece of fruit and sunflower seed crackers with dip	Oat cakes with hummus	Protein smoothie or shake	Homemade protein ball
Dinner	Celeriac with lentils	Almond sesame schnitzel	Steamed fish with greens	Healthy nachos with beans and guacamole	Fresh salmon patties	Vegetarian curry	Pastry-less quiche
Dessert (optional)	Berry watermelon sorbet	Fruit salad	'Chocolate' banana pot	Fruit salad	Baked egg custard	Berry watermelon sorbet	Lemon and date mousse
Before bed	1 glass water	1 glass water	1 glass water	1 glass water	1 glass water	1 glass water	1 glass water

Notes

SUPERFOODS FOR IVF

The term 'superfoods' refers to foods that are uniquely rich in micronutrients, vitamins, minerals and antioxidants. Antioxidants protect the body's cells from oxidation by free radical damage, thus helping prevent inflammation and disease. This is why antioxidant-dense foods are linked to numerous health benefits.

Many of the superfoods grow in especially challenging climates and conditions. In order to survive and thrive, they have developed protective phytonutrients (phytochemicals). These natural chemicals are also responsible for the nutrient-density of the food Mother Nature provides for us to eat.

What are free radicals?

It is important to know more about free radicals before reading further, as the benefits of many of these superfoods are often directly related to them. Free radicals are atoms or molecules that have too many or too few electrons, giving them a 'charge' and making them unstable. This means that inside the body they take or deposit electrons, which damage the cells in our body in the same way that an apple begins to turn brown if you leave half of it uneaten for a while.

Free radicals come from both inside and outside of our bodies so we will always be exposed to them. However, it is exogenous free radicals (the ones from outside our bodies) that cause the greatest problems by putting excessive strain on our own antioxidant systems. So how can we defend ourselves from free radicals?

Antioxidants inhibit the damage of cells by free radicals, so maximising our antioxidant intake through the food we eat (and, if required, supplements) can help reduce the amount of free radical damage that accumulates in our bodies as we get older.

Acai

Acai (pronounced ah-SAH-ee) is a great place to start as it has one of the highest oxygen radical absorption capacities (ORAC), which means it is really good at fighting free radicals. It is a little blue/purple berry that originates in the Amazon rainforest of Brazil. Considered to be one of the most powerful and nutritious superfoods on the planet, acai berries have been used for centuries for their legendary health and longevity-promoting properties. Acai is naturally high in essential fatty acids, amino acids (protein), dietary fibre and low in natural sugars. It is rich in vitamins and minerals especially beta-carotene, vitamin E, calcium and phosphorus. Acai is a great energy booster, beneficial for our cardiovascular, immune and nervous systems, skin health and muscle performance. It is best to use the freeze-dried form and add to smoothies.

Bee products:

Bell pollen

Bee pollen is one of nature's most nourishing and complete foods, as it contains almost all of the nutrients we need. Containing vitamin B9 (folate) and all essential amino acids, it is a delicious-tasting, energy-rich source of complete protein. Bee pollen is also full of anti-inflammatory properties and works wonders in addressing allergy symptoms as it reduces the presence of histamine. Its antimicrobial and antioxidant properties aid our immune systems and help to protect our cells against free radicals. In addition, bee pollen is rich in digestive-aiding enzymes, which enhance the body's ability to absorb nutrients from the food we eat.

Royal jelly

Royal jelly may help to support healthy hormone balance and egg quality. Royal jelly is the food that only the queen bee eats. It is rich in amino acids, vitamins, minerals, fatty acids and most importantly, protein. Royal jelly also contains acetylcholine, which is needed to transmit nerve messages from cell to cell. It should be taken for at least two months before IVF procedures begin and discontinued once your medication is started.

Caution: If you are allergic or think you are allergic to bees or bee products, do not take royal jelly or bee propolis.

Cacao

Cacao (pronounced ka-kow) beans are the seeds of an Amazonian fruiting tree and source of all chocolate and cocoa products. As the temperature is never allowed to exceed 40°C, the powder is considered a 'raw' food with all heat-sensitive vitamins such as iron, minerals such as magnesium, and antioxidants remaining intact, thereby maximising digestion and absorption. In fact, cacao has over 360 per cent more antioxidants than regular cocoa! It is one of nature's finest superfoods. It is beneficial for mood health as it contains naturally occurring phytochemicals like theobromine (considered an aphrodisiac), phenylethylamine (released when we fall in love), and anandamide (the 'bliss' chemical). Like all superfoods, cacao straddles the line between a food and a beneficial medicine.

Cacao is rich in flavour, and a little goes a long way. It is considered to have approximately 1 per cent caffeine (as compared to tea at 4 per cent and coffee which can be more than 10 per cent) so it is an exception to the 'avoid caffeine' recommendation!

Carob

Carob is made from the fruit pods of a large tropical leguminous evergreen tree. Originating in Egypt, carob has been enjoyed as a natural sweetener for at least 4,000 years, before sugar itself was introduced. In fact, the Greeks called carob 'Egyptian fig' due to its natural sweet taste. The pods are ground into a sweet, fine powder, while the seeds are used to make locust bean gum thickener. Carob is a source of dietary fibre, calcium, iron, potassium, magnesium, manganese, copper, vitamin B2, amino acids (protein) and antioxidants.

Chia seeds

Chia seeds are packed full of goodness, containing essential fatty acids and protein. They make a nice addition to smoothies, salads and porridge. They are also a great raw egg substitute when making home-made sorbets (it is important to avoid raw egg in pregnancy due to possible salmonella poisoning).

Chlorella

Chlorella comes from algae and is popular due to its high protein and nutrient content. Its benefits include aiding digestion and boosting energy and mood due to its high magnesium content. Chlorella stimulates probiotic growth and absorbs toxins in the intestine, which helps prevent constipation and stop toxic material, including metals like mercury, from being reabsorbed into the bloodstream. The taste is not to everyone's liking, so consider taking this in a tablet form.

Coconut

Coconut in its many forms has had quite a health revival. Its water and oil have been making their mark in the 'clean diet' market in recent times. Coconut milk, cream and fresh young coconut flesh are also popular. Coconut contains medium-chain saturated fatty acids which support the health of the immune system, thyroid gland, nervous system and skin, and provide fast energy. Coconuts also help support healthy hormone production and regulate blood sugar levels. It also contains lauric acid (a powerful anti-viral substance), making it an effective antimicrobial agent. Coconut helps the body use good fats more effectively. Coconut oil and omega-3 fatty acids are twice as effective when taken together as when taken alone.

Dulse

Dulse seaweed is a natural treasure chest of goodness, with vitamins A, B1, B2, B3, B6, B12, C, and E, and minerals like potassium, calcium, magnesium, phosphorous, chromium, iodine and zinc and trace elements. Sea vegetables are alkalising and contain 10 to 20 times *more* bioavailable minerals (especially iodine) and vitamins than land vegetables. A lack of iodine can contribute to thyroid gland problems. Enjoy dulse in soups, stocks, stews, miso, stir-fries or savoury dishes.

Hemp seeds

Hemp seeds are one of the most nutritional seeds on offer. Hemp seeds are a complete protein source, which means they contain all of the essential amino acids our bodies need. They also have a great balance of vitamins, enzymes and an ideal ratio of essential fats and polyunsaturated fatty acids, unlike any other superfood. These fats are important for hormone, skin, hair and overall health. Hemp can be consumed as seeds, oil and milk or ground up as a protein powder. These seeds help lower cholesterol, blood pressure and inflammation; boost and sustain energy; and are of benefit to our circulatory and immune systems.

Goji berries

These antioxidant-rich blue-red super berries are perhaps the most nutritionally rich berry on earth. They are a complete protein source (on par with bee pollen) and contain an abundance of minerals and vitamins including vitamins A and E. Known for their longevity properties, enhancing libido and sexual function, goji berries also enhance the immune system, repair skin damage (and keep your youthful glow!), strengthen the adrenal glands, support liver function, and increase alkalinity (good for addressing inflammation) and vitality.

Goji berries are found more commonly in their dried form to protect them in transit, but also as extract powder, juice, liquid tincture and oil (for topical skincare). They taste delicious sprinkled on top of porridge or salads.

Lucuma

Lucuma is a South American fruit and a source of beta-carotene (which gives the fruit its bright orange colour), vitamin B3 (a mood-boosting vitamin), iron, calcium, phosphorus and zinc. The powdered form is often used as a natural sweetener thanks to its caramel-like flavour. It is a delicious way of adding amino acids (protein), fibre, vitamins and minerals to smoothies and desserts – although cooking will lower the nutritional concentration, so it is best used in uncooked recipes such as smoothies. It is a popular ice-cream flavour in South America. Despite being sweet, lucuma is lower on the glycemic index, making it a healthier choice for sugar-sensitive people.

Maca

Maca is a tuber vegetable that grows in the Andean Mountains of Peru. It has 2,000 years of traditional use for its hormone-balancing and libido-boosting effects. Also known as the 'Peruvian ginseng', maca helps increase energy and stamina and is a wonderful fertility superfood. Like most superfoods, maca is a source of complex carbohydrates, dietary fibre, protein vitamins and minerals.

As a natural adaptogen, maca helps the body cope with stress. It helps balance hormones, yet it does not contain any hormones itself. Maca does this by nourishing and balancing the endocrine (hormone) system. This balance is important in preparing for IVF because a healthy hormone balance contributes to healthier eggs. Maca is also a great mood balancer so it is the perfect thing to add to your breakfast porridge or warm drink if you wake up feeling a cranky or premenstrual. Many people experience a noticeable difference in energy after just a few days.

Maqui

Maqui (pronounced 'mah-key') is the 'Patagonian super fruit'. With a deep purple colour and mild berry taste, it is native to Chile and has a long history of use for longevity and improving strength. With an ORAC antioxidant score that's three times higher than the acai berry, it contains antioxidants (anthocyanins – also found in blueberries), vitamins A and C, iron, potassium and omega oil. Add to smoothies, yoghurt, cereal or porridge, salad dressings, or even your water bottle.

Moringa

The moringa tree is known as the 'miracle tree' due to its medicinal properties. Made up of almost 25 per cent protein, it contains all nine essential amino acids. It also has an exceptionally high ORAC rating. Moringa comes in a powder form and is great for giving an energy boost to your smoothies. It is an excellent superfood to consider for anyone struggling with fatigue or iron deficiency.

Spirulina

Spirulina is made from blue-green algae just like chlorella. Known as the 'protein queen', spirulina contains the highest concentration of protein found in any food. It also contains an array of nutrients including chlorophyll, vitamins, minerals, essential fatty acids (GLA in particular), nucleic acids and a spectrum of antioxidants.

Spirulina encourages the growth of healthy gut bacterial flora, benefiting digestion and helping prevent candida overgrowth. It is also a blood builder due to its high iron content (as much as you would get from eating red meat). Not only is spirulina highly digestible but it also helps the body to absorb minerals, lowers cholesterol and protects the immune system. Just like chlorella, spirulina has a really strong flavour, so many people prefer to take it in tablet form. If you would like to add it to a smoothie, start with just half a teaspoon or so until you get used to the taste.

Wheatgrass

Wheatgrass is an excellent alkaliser and has properties very similar to our own blood, making it a great superfood to increase vitality and for helping us look and feel young! It also cleanses the blood, organs and lymphatic system by helping to eliminate toxins. With twice the amount of vitamin A as carrots, more vitamin C than oranges, a full spectrum of B vitamins, wheatgrass really is a nutrient powerhouse. It also contains all of the essential amino acids, making it a complete, easily digestible protein source.

N.B. Although wheatgrass is normally gluten-free, there is the possibility that it could be contaminated with gluten during the harvesting process.

How to enjoy superfoods

There are many superfood brands to try and the best thing to do is find a brand you love. Look in your local health food store, browse online and stock your cupboards with these amazing superfoods and powders to help nourish your body.

Here are some ways you can enjoy superfoods:

- Mix a teaspoon or two into smoothies, sprinkle on your breakfast cereal (hot or cold), or yoghurt.
- Use in baked goods like gluten-free bread, muffins or homemade granola.
- Mix into raw desserts or use to flavour roasted nuts and seeds.
- Make into protein balls.
- Blend into hot drinks like tea, or as a hot chocolate replacement.
- Use to flavour homemade nut milks.
- Add to sauces and marinades.

For delicious and inspiring superfood recipes, please refer to the companion *IVF Diet Cookbook*.

TRADITIONAL CHINESE MEDICINE, FERTILITY & DIET

Traditional Chinese Medicine (TCM) practitioners and acupuncturists may provide you dietary advice based on your TCM body type.

As with everything in TCM, food categories affect the '*yin-yang*' balance. Foods can be divided into Hot, Cold, Warm and Cool, commonly known as the 'four natures'.

Every food is viewed as having *yin, yang* or neutral properties. *Yang* foods are warming, stimulating and dry, whereas *yin* foods are cooling, calming and wet. There are various neutral foods that share the characteristics of both. Different foods may be added to or eliminated in your diet, depending on your TCM type.

Warming *yang* foods are eaten more often during the cold months of the year; cooling *yin* goods during the heat of summer. The warming or cooling effects derive from the nature of the food and the herbs and spices they are cooked with, rather than the temperature at which they are served.

Yin foods

Cool and cold foods are said to be *yin* foods. These foods are used to clear heat and eliminate toxins. Generally speaking, the sweeter the food, the more *yin* energy it holds. Fruits and vegetables tend to be *yin*. This reflects cooking methods too: yin methods are light, fast and keep the nutrients intact, such as steaming, sautéing and stir-frying.

Yang foods

Warm and hot foods are said to be *yang* foods. These foods are used to expel cold. *Yang* foods tend to be saltier and more savoury. Meat and animal products are often yang (though fish and eggs are neutral). *Yang*-style cooking methods include stewing, slow-cooking, baking and roasting.

Other TCM tips

- Eat regularly to avoid getting hungry.
- Avoid eating in excess.
- Don't eat late at night.
- Eat slowly and eat with awareness (e.g. not in front of the television!)
- Avoid icy cold drinks.
- Avoid spicy foods.

Section 5

Supplements & Herbal Medicines

This section examines some of the supplements and herbal medicines you can take during your IVF journey.

Notes

SUPPLEMENTS

There is ample scientific evidence and clinical proof to support the use of nutritional supplements before, during and after the IVF cycle.

Although you could look at the comprehensive list below and think to yourself you could benefit from every single supplement, it is a good idea to have a naturopath, nutritionist or doctor trained in integrative medicine to prescribe what is most indicated for your needs.

What's more, it is advisable to find a naturopath or nutritionist who specialises in infertility and IVF support. They will have a deep understanding of IVF, can read your hormone blood tests to understand your situation, and can support you during critical times such as egg retrieval, embryo transfer and directly post-transfer.

It is a good idea to provide your naturopath with a copy of your IVF treatment protocol so he/she can more accurately plan your naturopathic support treatment.

Below is a list of supplements recommended for all or different stages of the IVF process. Don't be overwhelmed by the list, many of the nutrients can be found in a comprehensive prenatal vitamin and mineral supplement. Your naturopath or nutritionist will not only prescribe what is important for you but also additional doses if required.

Alpha lipoic acid

Alpha lipoic acid is the only antioxidant that works on the shell and inside the egg. It enhances fertilisation, improves egg penetration by sperm and implantation rates, and reduces the risk of implantation loss.[20] Every mature woman should take this!

[20] Ruder EH, Hartman TJ, Blumberg J, Goldman MB. Oxidative stress and antioxidants; exposure and impact on female fertility Hum Reprod Update 2008: Jul-Aug;14(4):345-57. Epub 2008 Jun 4.

Food sources include meat, vegetables such as broccoli and spinach, and brewer's yeast. Recommended supplement dose is 300-600mcg per day.

Beta carotene

Beta carotene is the vegetable precursor to vitamin A. It plays an important role in egg maturation and function. High levels correlate with strong progesterone levels. Food sources include yellow or deep orange fruit and vegetables like cantaloupe and butternut squash, and dark green leafy vegetables like spinach. Recommended supplement dose: 10-30mg per day.

Bioflavanoids

Bioflavanoids are found in nature with vitamin C and assist uterine blood flow. Food sources include citrus fruits, blackcurrants and buckwheat. Recommended supplement dose is 1000-1500mg per day (often combined with vitamin C).

Calcium

Calcium signalling is required for egg maturation and fertilisation. Food sources include dairy products, green leafy vegetables, broccoli, okra, oily fish (mackerel, salmon, sardines), molasses, bone meal (and broth), nuts and seeds, especially sesame seeds. Recommended supplement is dose 1000-1500mg per day (evening dose is preferred as calcium uptake is greatest at rest).

Chromium

Chromium improves glucose tolerance where fertility is impaired due to insulin resistance or obesity. Food sources include wholegrains, brewer's yeast, broccoli, potatoes, green beans, mushrooms, grapes and raisins. Recommended supplement dose is 100mcg-400mcg, and up to1200mcg per day if obese.

Coenzyme Q10 (CoQ10)

Coenzyme Q10 (CoQ10) is another powerful antioxidant required for both egg and sperm health. It has been shown to improve egg quality (working inside the egg) and fertilisation rates.[21] Food sources include spinach, tuna, sardines and beef. Recommended supplement dose is 100-600mg per day for at least three months.

Women less than 30 years: 100mg per day; 30-38 years: 300mg per day; 38 years plus: up to 600mg per day. For older women and those with a history of miscarriage, continue to take 300mg per day in the first month of the first trimester, then 150mg for the remaining two months of the first trimester.

There are two forms of CoQ10 - ubiquinone and ubiquinol. CoQ10 starts off as ubiquinone and then is converted within the cell to the more powerful ubiquinol. As a woman ages, her body's ability to convert ubiquinone to ubiquinol declines. Ubiquinol is the most biologically active form of coenzyme Q10 and does not need to be converted by the body. Ubiquinol is eight times more potent than ubiquinone and supplementation leads to higher blood levels in older women.

However, if ubiquinone is the only form you can obtain, it will still provide the much-needed antioxidant support required for egg quality.

[21] Yaakov Bentov. The use of mitochondrial nutrition to improve the outcome of infertility treatment in older patients. Fertility and Sterility. Volume 93, Issue 1, Pages 272-275, 1 January 2010.

DHEA

DHEA (dehydroepiandrosterone) is shown to rejuvenate ovarian function and improve ovarian reserve and progesterone levels.[22]

It is highly indicted for poor IVF responders.[23] It is a steroid precursor hormone produced in the adrenal glands and required for hormone production. It is also used to assist vitality and libido. Recommended supplement dose is 25-75mg per day for a minimum of three months, especially if aged 40 plus.

Note: PCOS patients should be cautious (watch for conversion to testosterone, especially if low in vitamin D and zinc; 7-keto form is preferred).

DHEA supplementation may benefit women undergoing IVF treatment

Several study results indicate that supplementation with 25mg of DHEA three times a day may exert a beneficial effect on ovarian reserves (low AMH readings), improve embryo quality and produce a significantly higher live birth rate for poor-responder patients on IVF treatment compared with the control group.

Addition of DHEA for poor-responder patients before and during IVF treatment improves the pregnancy rate: A randomized prospective study, Wiser A, Shulman A, et al, Hum Reprod, 2010 Aug 21; [Epub ahead of print].

Impact of DHEA on clinical outcome in poor responders: A pilot study in women undergoing in vitro fertilization, using bologna criteria. Journal of Reproductive Sciences, 2014; Vol 7; Issue 3: 175-180

[22] DHEA supplementation increases baseline follicular phase progesterone levels," Weissman A, Horowitz E, et al, Gynecol Endocrinol, 2011 April 18; [Epub ahead of print]. (Address: Department of Obstetrics and Gynecology, IVF Unit, Edith Wolfson Medical Center, Holon, and Sackler Faculty of Medicine, Tel Aviv University, Tel Aviv, Israel

[23] DHEA supplementation improves follicular microenvironment in poor responder patients," Artini PG, Simi G, et al, Gynecol Endocrinol, 2012 Jul 26; [Epub ahead of print]. (Address: Paolo Giovanni Artini, Department of Reproductive Medicine and Child Development, Division of Obstetrics and Gynaecology, University of Pisa, Pisa, Italy.

Inositol

Inositol is a type of B vitamin that aids in reversing insulin resistance, stabilising glucose levels and improving ovarian function. Food sources include wholegrains, citrus fruits, brewer's yeast, unrefined molasses and lecithin. Recommended supplement dose may vary from 200-500mg per day. (Refer to Myo-inositol in this chapter for more information.)

Iodine

Iodine is required for thyroid function, follicle development and maturation of eggs. It is crucial in pregnancy for the development of the baby's brain. Food sources include fish, shellfish, kelp and other sea vegetables (arame, kombu, nori and wakame) and dairy products.

Although there are some doctors and authors promoting iodine as the 'cure all' for thyroid disorders, it is important not to self-prescribe higher doses than what may be found in a prenatal supplement without guidance from your doctor or naturopath. Iodine supplementation is controversial in cases of low selenium levels as it may induce hyperthyroidism. Do not exceed 300mcg per day, unless otherwise prescribed by your doctor or naturopath.

Women who have thyroid disease or take thyroid medication should consult their doctor or naturopath before taking iodine supplements. Iodine should not be taken at the same time of the day as iron.

Iron

Iron forms oxygen-carrying red blood cells. A deficiency contributes to a lack of ovulation, infertility and serious problems in pregnancy. Other deficiency signs and symptoms include fatigue, low mood, hair loss and decreased resistance to infections. Food sources include red meat, chicken, eggs, pulses, dark green leafy vegetables, dried apricots and prunes, seeds and molasses.

Before taking iron supplements, ask your doctor for a blood test to check your iron status - ferritin should ideally be above 40-50. It is necessary to address low levels of iron before embarking on an IVF cycle. If levels are low, the embryo is less likely to implant (low ferritin can add to poor uterine circulation in cases of a thin uterine lining, especially in those patients with good oestrogen levels). Recommended supplement dose is 12-24mg elemental iron per day based on results (take a non-constipating form such as a bioavailable amino acid chelate - bisglycinate form). Take with vitamin C and away from tea, calcium and zinc (the exception is when it is all combined in a prenatal formula). Iron is best taken on an empty stomach first thing in the morning, at least 20 minutes before food.

L-Arginine

L-Arginine is mainly indicated for poor IVF responders as it may increase the number of mature follicles and improve uterine receptivity. Food sources include red meat, nuts, spinach, lentils, wholegrains, seafood and eggs. Recommended supplement dose is 2-16g per day (usual dose is 2g twice daily). Some women may not respond. Be guided by your doctor or naturopath.

Note: L-Arginine should not be taken if you have herpes as it can trigger an outbreak. If it's a mild case, you can counter this with lysine.

L-Carnitine

L-Carnitine improves egg quality (more specifically, the fluid, DNA arrangement and oxygen utilisation of egg). L-Carnitine has shown better results than L-arginine with regards to egg quality. Food sources include meat, dairy, fish, chicken, avocado, wholegrains and asparagus. Recommended supplement dose is 4g per day.

Magnesium

Magnesium is critical for the health of the adrenal and nervous systems and overall stress management. Low levels may be implicated in hormonal irregularities and miscarriage. Up to 80 per cent of the population have some degree of magnesium deficiency. Food sources include green leafy vegetables, wholegrains, seafood and nuts, especially almonds, seeds and molasses. Recommended supplement dose is 500-1000mg per day.

Melatonin

Melatonin improves responsiveness to IVF and egg quality.[24] It is also recommended for all older women undergoing IVF. Studies also confirm melatonin is likely to improve embryo quality in women undergoing IVF or ICSI.[25] It is an antioxidant and a hormone that is activated when night time falls and helps us sleep. Some foods that promote the production of melatonin include cherries, oats, bananas, rice, tomatoes and oats. Recommended supplement dose is 2-6mg per day (be guided by your doctor or naturopath as the dose is weight dependant). Take as low a dose as possible. Take away from thyroxine (which is usually a morning dose); preferably at night since it is a sleep hormone, which also help with sleep problems.

[24] www.ovarianresearch.com/content/5/1/5 Tamura et al. Journal of Ovarian Research 2012, 5:5

[25] Gynecol Endocrinol. 2012 Feb;28(2):91-3. doi: 10.3109/09513590.2011.589925. Epub 2011 Jul 20. The efficacy of melatonin administration on oocyte quality. Batıoğlu AS1, Sahin U, Gürlek B, Oztürk N, Unsal E.

Supporting Studies: Can Melatonin Boost Egg and Embryo Quality?

1. A 2014 study published in *Gynaecology and Endocrinology* looked at women who were prescribed 3mg of melatonin nightly for at least two weeks prior to IVF. The researchers compared outcomes for women who underwent two treatment cycles, the first with no melatonin and the second with melatonin treatment.

For women whose embryos had poor fertilisation rates in the first cycle, there was a dramatic increase in fertilisation rates after melatonin treatment (35.1 per cent versus 68.2 per cent). Also, the rate of good quality embryos increased from 48 per cent to 65.6 per cent. The study concluded that oral melatonin supplementation can have a beneficial effect on the improvement of fertilisation and embryo quality due to a reduction in oxidative damage.[26]

2. A 2011 study analysed the effect of melatonin in women with sleep disturbances. Sixty women were randomised to receive melatonin or no treatment prior to IVF. Although sleep status remained roughly the same, melatonin-treated women had significantly more eggs retrieved of greater quality. The study concluded that IVF patients with sleep disorders may benefit from melatonin administration in improving egg and the embryo quality.[27]

Melatonin treatment in the three months prior to IVF is recommended by some of the top fertility clinics in the US, especially for women who are classed as 'poor responders.' This is

[26] Gynecol Endocrinol. 2014 May;30(5):359-62. doi: 10.3109/09513590.2013.879856. Epub 2014 Mar 17. Oral melatonin supplementation improves oocyte and embryo quality in women undergoing in vitro fertilization-embryo transfer. Nishihara T1, Hashimoto S, Ito K, Nakaoka Y, Matsumoto K, Hosoi Y, Morimoto Y.

[27] J Assist Reprod Genet. 2011 Sep;28(9):815-20. doi: 10.1007/s10815-011-9604-y. Epub 2011 Jul 12. Melatonin improves the oocyte and the embryo in IVF patients with sleep disturbances but does not improve the sleeping problems. Eryilmaz OG1, Devran A, Sarikaya E, Aksakal FN, Mollamahmutoğlu L, Cicek N.

more evidence that melatonin is a 'superstar' fertility supplement that may help maximise your chance of IVF success.

Myo-inositol

Myo-inositol (also sold as D-chiro-inositol) is indicated for healthy ovulation, hormone balancing, and improving egg quality and development. It also supports insulin control, stabilising blood sugar levels and supporting androgen dominance in those with ovarian issues such as PCOS. Myo-inositol is a natural nutrient belonging to the vitamin B group. As the second messenger of serotonin, myo-inositol has also shown some success in PMS mood support.[28]

Recommended dose as per successful clinical trials is 2g twice per day.

> Myo-inositol and melatonin improve ovarian stimulation and pregnancy outcomes in women with infertility and poor oocyte quality
>
> In a study involving 46 women who failed to conceive in previous IVF cycles due to poor egg quality, supplementation with myo-inositol (4 g/d) and melatonin (3 mg/d) for a period of three months, followed by another IVF cycle, was found to be associated with improved ovarian stimulation and pregnancy outcomes (13 pregnancies occurred, nine confirmed, four evolved in spontaneous abortion). The number of mature eggs, the fertilisation rate and the number of both total and top-quality embryos transferred were statistically higher, compared to the previous IVF cycle. These results suggest that supplementation with myo-inositol and melatonin may be of benefit to women undergoing IVF deemed to have poor egg quality.

[28] Rizzo P, RaffoneE, Benedetto V. EurRev Med PharmacolSci. 2010 Jun;14(6):555-61. Ciotta L, et al. EurRev Med PharmacolSci. 2011 May;15(5):509-14. PapaleoE, et al. FertilSteril. 2009 May;91(5):1750-4.

NAC (N-acetyl cysteine)

NAC (N-acetyl cysteine) is an antioxidant that improves ovarian function and insulin sensitivity. It is also indicated for PCOS, diabetes and elevated homocysteine levels. Since it is an amino acid, most protein foods will contain it. Recommended supplement dose is 1200-1800mg per day. Take with food in a divided dose to avoid nausea.

Omega 3 EPA/DHA oils

Omega 3 EPA/DHA oils improve uterine blood flow and may help prevent miscarriage (can be effective as aspirin). They are also necessary for the proper development of a baby's brain and nervous system. In addition, they are important for hormone balance, thyroid health and overall cell quality.

Food sources include oily fish (herring, mackerel, mullet, sardines and salmon) and flaxseeds. Recommended supplement dose is 4000mg per day providing 795mg DHA, 1190mg EPA from quality, non-contaminated pure fish oil.

If you are taking blood-thinning medication (for example, aspirin or clexane), you should not increase omega 3 intake without first checking with your doctor or naturopath as omega 3 can also thin the blood.

PQQ

PQQ (Pyrroloquinoline quinine) is a novel vitamin-like compound found in plant foods that is showing a wide range of benefits including improved egg quality. The best food source is natto, a pungent Japanese dish of fermented soybeans. If natto isn't to your liking, PQQ is also found in parsley, green tea, green peppers, kiwi fruit and papaya. Recommended supplement dose is 10-20mg per day. PQQ appears to be a good complement to other supplements that support cellular function, such as CoQ10 and alpha-lipoic acid.

Is PQQ the next nutrient superstar?

PQQ has been known since 1979 but a team in Japan has now declared it a vitamin - the first new vitamin to be discovered since vitamin B12 in 1948. It is likely to be considered an essential nutrient in the future.

Medical research indicates that PQQ is a powerful antioxidant, and it helps to preserve the energy-producing units of your cells. Due to this effect, it may well be the next 'fountain of youth'. Apart from its researched use on fertility and egg quality, other reported medical benefits include the prevention of heart attacks, strokes, cancer, osteoporosis, obesity and intestinal disease. Several clinical trials are either completed, waiting publication or are in process.

Pre-natal multivitamins

A pre-natal multivitamin will usually contain everything listed above and for some women, this may be sufficient.

Multivitamin supplementation improves nutritional status in women undergoing IVF

Studies involving women undergoing IVF who supplemented with a prenatal multivitamin and mineral supplement were found to have normalised levels of trace elements in blood and follicular fluid (fluid in and around the egg), lower oxidative stress and improved antioxidant levels compared to control groups.

'Multivitamin and mineral supplementation modulates oxidative stress and antioxidant vitamin levels in serum and follicular fluid of women undergoing in vitro fertilization,' Ozkaya MO, Naziroglu M, Fertil Steril, 2010 Nov; 94(6): 2465-6.
'Effects of multivitamin/mineral supplementation on trace element levels in serum and follicular fluid of women undergoing in vitro fertilization (IVF),' Ozkaya MO, Naziroglu M, et al, Biol Trace Elem Res, 2011 Jan; 139(1): 1-9.

Probiotics

Alterations to vaginal flora are linked to failure to conceive, miscarriage and preterm birth. Probiotics are important for immune and digestive health. Food sources include live yoghurt and fermented foods. Recommended supplement dose is 25-50 x10(9) organisms for two to three months to restore balance. Also consider Saccharomyces boulardii with a probiotic to reset bowel flora, especially if you suffer from irritable bowel syndrome (IBS) and candida.

Selenium

Selenium deficiency is strongly associated with recurrent miscarriage. It is a potent antioxidant protecting developing eggs and the embryo(s) from free radical damage. It is also essential for thyroid health. Food sources include Brazil nuts, seafood, eggs, garlic, the onion family, asparagus, broccoli and mushrooms. Recommended supplement dose is 200-300mcg per day.

Vitamin B complex

Embryonic development depends on all B vitamins. Food sources include wholegrains, brewer's yeast, seeds, nuts, eggs, yoghurt, fruits, meats, leafy vegetables and intestinal bacteria. Recommended supplement dose: 50-100mg of an activated B complex is preferred per day. If there is a history of miscarriage and/or stress, take a higher dose.

Vitamin B6

Vitamin B6 supports the luteal phase and progesterone levels by increasing the brain chemicals serotonin and dopamine, which control FSH and LH. It supports a healthy uterine lining, reduces homocysteine (high levels of this amino acid are associated with poor egg and embryo quality), protects against miscarriage, and reduces prolactin levels. Food sources include poultry, fish, bananas, leafy green vegetables such as spinach, potatoes, chickpeas, lentils and oats. Recommended supplement dose: 50mg of an activated B6 form is preferred. If there is a history of miscarriage, take a higher dose.

Vitamin B9

Vitamin B9 (also known as folate) supports egg quality and maturation, reduces homocysteine levels and improves DNA methylation, assisting egg and early embryo quality. It also helps prevent against placenta abnormalities and neural tube defects. Food sources include leafy greens such as spinach and turnip greens, pulses, wholegrains and oats. Recommended supplement dose: take up to 4000mcg per day if there is a history of spina bifida. If a high homocysteine level is an issue, take with vitamins B6 and B12. For a MTHFR genetic mutation, take a bioactive form – for heterozygous: 500 mcg as Calcium Folinate and 500 mcg as L-5-Methyltetrahydrofolate (5-MTHFR); or 1mg 5-MTHFR form if homozygous.

Vitamin B12

Vitamin B12 is required for healthy gene regulation, DNA and RNA synthesis, and regular ovulation. Deficiency is linked to infertility and recurrent miscarriages (especially in older women). It works with folate to prevent neural tube defects. Food sources include animal protein such as meat and chicken, fish, dairy and eggs. Recommended supplement dose may vary from 800-2000mcg per day. If you have been taking folate on its own, ask your doctor/naturopath to rule out B12 anaemia as this is common after being on folate alone for a long time. The type of B12 used will depend on genetics and ethnicity e.g. eastern Europeans need a high absorbable form such as a sublingual dose.

Vitamin C

Vitamin C is important for regular ovulation. It works with vitamin E to protect developing and maturing eggs from free radical damage. It also helps with implantation by working on growth and repair of the follicles and uterine lining. In addition, it assists with progesterone support. Food sources include citrus fruits, cherries, kiwi fruit, guava, cantaloupe, strawberries, potatoes, red peppers (capsicum), tomatoes, cruciferous vegetables and peas. Recommended supplement dose is 500mg to 5000mg per day (divided dose). Avoid or limit if you are amine sensitive.

Vitamin D (D3)

Known as the sunshine vitamin, vitamin D (D3) is important for genetic health, embryo implantation, immunity and bone health. Higher levels of vitamin D have been found in successful IVF pregnancy rates.[29] It is especially important for the first trimester of pregnancy as it is involved in cell replication and assists the mother's immune system to maintain pregnancy.[30] It also promotes normal skeletal and brain development in the developing baby. It is indicated for a history of miscarriage and low AMH levels.

We get most of our vitamin D from the action of sunlight on our skin. Natural food sources include eggs, fortified food, oily fish such as salmon, sardines, herring, mackerel and tuna, and very small amounts in beef liver, cheese and egg yolk.

Recommended supplement dose: 1000IU per day of D3 - cholecalciferol (better absorbed than D2) as a minimum but may be as high as 10,000IU per day in severe deficiency states (especially if you live above latitude 40 degrees north, or below latitude 40 degrees south) but be guided by your doctor or naturopath.

[29] Ozkan S et.al Replete vitamin D stores predict reproductive success following in vitro fertilisation. Fertil Steril. 2010 Sep; 94(4): 1314-9.
[30] Nutrients 2012, 4, 799-840;

Some practitioners suggest 10,000IU per day for one month, then 5000IU per day for the next two months. Re-test at the end of three months. Others prescribe 50,000IU of vitamin D once a week for eight weeks (in most patients' blood levels will rise on average by 100 per cent).

There's a widely held belief that in sunny climates such as Australia and New Zealand and warmer parts of the US, people should have all the vitamin D they need - but the reality is one in three people are deficient. This is largely attributed to people using sunscreen with a high SPF factor which is great to prevent melanoma, but unfortunately reduces our ability to convert 7-dehydrocholesterol into cholecalciferol. Office and shift workers also miss out because they're commuting before the sun comes out and heading home as it sets. Try getting out in the sun for even just 10 minutes a day, ensuring skin is free from sunscreen (you can wear a hat). Other factors which affect conversion are ageing and chemicals such as sodium lauryl sulphate (present in skin washes, bubble baths, mineral body lotions, fake tans and body scrubs). The decline in the body's ability to synthesise vitamin D through the skin starts at 20, and by the time we're 50 it has halved.

Vitamin E

Vitamin E is an essential fertility vitamin. It is a potent antioxidant and helps to reduce oxidative damage, maintain the health of the ovaries, regulate hormone levels, assist uterine blood circulation and support lining, and prevent 'sticky blood'. Food sources include eggs, wheatgerm, molasses, sweet potato, leafy vegetables, nuts and seeds. Recommended supplement dose range: 400-2000IU divided dose per day. With vitamin E supplements, the lower the dose, the more you absorb, so it is best to divide the dose e.g.500IU twice daily.

Vitamin K2

Vitamin K2 is indicated for blood coagulation or clotting disorders. It can be taken throughout pregnancy as well. Food sources include green leafy vegetables, egg yolk, molasses, cauliflower and natto. Recommended supplement dose: 50-100mcg per day unless otherwise prescribed (much higher doses may be prescribed).

Zinc

Zinc is important for gene regularity hormones and is crucial for synthesising DNA and the receptor proteins for oestrogen, progesterone and testosterone. A deficiency can alter pituitary hormone (FSH and LH) levels, may cause abnormal egg development, delay ovulation and increase the risk of miscarriage. It is also essential for thyroid health. Food sources include oysters (highest source), seafood, meat, turkey, wholegrains, mushrooms, eggs, sunflower and pumpkin seeds (pepitas). Recommended supplement dose is 40-80mg per day.

Supplements for PCOS

Many women with PCOS are diagnosed as being 'Clomid-resistant' when their ovaries refuse to respond to stimulation by clomiphene citrate (clomid). Such women are often hastened to try stronger ovarian-stimulating medications - or IVF - but a simple, inexpensive and lesser-known treatment may help.

NAC is an antioxidant which is being increasingly studied in PCOS women and shows promise as a novel way to improve the ovulation response to Clomid. NAC has been shown to improve insulin sensitivity, decrease androgen levels and may help a PCOS woman to ovulate without resorting to IVF. It is safe and well tolerated. Varying doses from 1200mg (1.2g) to 3000mg (3g) (if obese) may be given alongside clomid for five days beginning on day 3 of the cycle.[31]

NAC (at 1200mg per day) when combined with L-arginine (at 1600mg per day) has also been shown in studies to restore healthy ovarian function and improve insulin sensitivity in PCOS patients.[32]

If you are not responding well to Clomid and not quite ready to consider IVF, ask your doctor or naturopath about taking NAC (with or without L-Arginine) alongside Clomid on your next cycle.

Other natural supplements with equally impressive effects on PCOS include myo-inositol, DIM, chromium, magnesium and vitamin D. For more information on natural support for PCOS, please refer to my book, *'The Natural PCOS Diet'* jennyblondel.com.

In summary

This is an exhaustive list of nutritional supplements. You may benefit from just a few, to several listed above. Be guided by your naturopath, nutritionist and/or doctor as to the most appropriate supplements to complement your IVF protocol.

[31] Acta Obstet Gynecol Scand. 2007;86(2):218-22. NAC and clomiphene citrate for induction of ovulation in polycystic ovary syndrome: a cross-over trial. Badawy A, State O, Abdelgawad S.

[32] J Endocrinol Invest. 2009 Dec;32(11):870-2. Epub 2009 Apr 15. Prolonged treatment with NAC and L-arginine restores gonadal function in patients with polycystic ovary syndrome. Masha A, et al.

Notes

HERBAL MEDICINES

The use of herbs in preparation for IVF

Herbal remedies can be used to help prepare your body and optimise your health in the months preceding an IVF cycle. There are some herbs that cannot be co-prescribed; however, there are some key herbs to assist with stress management, immune health and hormone balancing.

Find a naturopath or medical herbalist who specialises in infertility and IVF support. They will have a deeper understanding of IVF, can decipher your hormone blood tests, and support you during critical times such as egg retrieval, embryo transfer and directly post-transfer.

Once again, it is a good idea to provide your naturopath or medical herbalist with a copy of your IVF treatment protocol so he/she can more accurately plan your naturopathic support treatment.

Herbal medicine for fertility support

Herbal medicine has existed for as long as there have been plants growing on our planet.

There are many effective herbs to help regulate hormones and address conditions such as PCOS, endometriosis, amenorrhoea, fibroids, irregular cycles and history of miscarriage. There are also some excellent herbs to help support the stress response.

Here is a list of just a few herbs that may be used before an IVF cycle:

- Hormone balancing herbs: Black cohosh, Peony, Licorice, Wild yam, Chaste tree (Vitex agnus castus), Dong quai and Tribulus
- Herbs to support threatened miscarriage: False unicorn root, Dong quai, Peony and Shatavari

- Adrenal (stress supporting) herbs: Kava, Licorice, Rehmannia, Rhodiola, Siberian ginseng and Withania
- Blood sugar-regulating herbs: Gymnema and Cinnamon
- Liver-supporting herbs: Bupleurum, Dandelion root, Milk thistle, Rosemary and Schizandra
- Immune-modulating herbs: Echinacea, Hemidesmus and Rehmannia
- Other herbs that may be indicated include Albizia, Baical skullcap, Coleus, Feverfew, Ginkgo biloba and Turmeric.

These herbs can be used in the months preceding and in preparation for the IVF cycle. But it is important to stop the hormone-balancing herbs once the ovarian stimulation (follicular) phase i.e. FSH injections begins. There are some cases where herbs such as False Unicorn Root are effective throughout an IVF procedure, especially in those with a history of miscarriage.

There are also other herbs that can be used safely in conjunction with IVF medications as they do not have any direct impact on the reproductive system. This is because they are supportive of the different systems that indirectly impact on overall fertility, for example, the use of Echinacea, Hemidesmus and Rehmannia for autoimmune system problems. Again, it is important that each individual situation be considered by your naturopath or medical herbalist when choosing which herbs to support you through the IVF process.

Better safe than sorry

Always consult a registered, experienced naturopath or medical herbalist about herbal medicine before or during an IVF cycle. Please never self-prescribe herbs. Self-administering herbs has the potential to lead to dosage problems, unwanted side effects and possible interactions.

IVF is not a procedure that comes without risks, regardless of whether you use herbal medicine or conventional medicine, or both. If you are committed to this path, make sure you are fully informed and understand how you can make your journey a safer experience.

It is also important to understand that more research needs to be conducted with regards to prescribing herbal medicine to assist the outcome of IVF.

Notes

SUPPLEMENTS FOR EACH PHASE OF IVF

Below is a guide for a potential supplement programme that may be of assistance during your IVF process. You may or may not require what is listed below, or you may require additional supplements and herbal medicine. Your naturopath or doctor will prescribe according to your requirements.

Supplements for preconception

- A good prenatal supplement preferably containing folate as a bioactive form
- Additional doses of supplements detailed in the previous chapter if deficient and advised by your naturopath
- Vitamin C
- Omega 3 EPA/DHA fish oil
- Alpha Lipoic acid
- Coenzyme Q10
- DHEA
- Melatonin
- Myo-inositol
- PQQ
- Probiotics
- Vitamin E.

Supplements for the follicular phase

- A good prenatal supplement preferably containing folate as a bioactive form
- Additional doses of supplements detailed in the previous chapter if deficient and advised by your naturopath
- Vitamin C
- Omega 3 EPA/DHA fish oil
- Alpha Lipoic acid

- Coenzyme Q10
- DHEA
- Melatonin
- Myo-inositol
- PQQ
- Probiotics
- Vitamin E.

No supplements for egg retrieval

You will need to stop all supplements 24 to 48 hours prior to egg retrieval and collection surgery. You may resume taking supplements 24 hours afterwards, with the exception of waiting a few more days before reintroducing Coenzyme Q10 and Omega 3 EPA/DHA fish oil.

Supplements for embryo transfer

Alongside dietary and lifestyle advice, you may also be prescribed some or all of the following supplements and herbal medicine depending on recommendations.

- A good prenatal supplement preferably containing folate as a bioactive form
- Additional doses of supplements detailed in the previous chapter if deficient and advised by your naturopath
- Vitamin C
- Omega 3 EPA/DHA fish oil
- Alpha Lipoic acid
- Coenzyme Q10
- Probiotics
- Vitamin E.

Your naturopath or medical herbalist may also prescribe some herbal medicine at this stage of treatment if required, such as immune-modulating herbal medicine including Hemidesmus and Rehmannia; and maybe False Unicorn Root if there is a history of miscarriage.

Supplements for luteal phase support

Continue with:

- A good prenatal supplement preferably containing folate as a bioactive form
- Additional doses of supplements detailed in the previous chapter if deficient and advised by your naturopath
- Vitamin C
- Alpha Lipoic acid
- Coenzyme Q10
- DHEA
- Melatonin
- PQQ
- Probiotics
- Vitamin E.

In addition to your prescribed progesterone support (injections, pessaries, gel - crinone), your naturopath may co-prescribe L-Arginine or L-Carnitine, Chaste tree and vitamin B6 to assist with uterine/endometrial lining thickness (especially if it is less than the ideal minimum of 7mm necessary for embryo implantation). Be guided by your doctor or naturopath.

Your naturopath or medical herbalist may also prescribe some immune-modulating herbs and uterine tonics such as False Unicorn Root at this stage of treatment.

Supplements for pregnancy

Refer to Section 9: When IVF Works – a dedicated section on pregnancy-related advice on diet and supplements.

Notes

Section 6

Other Holistic Therapies

There are a number of holistic therapies and lifestyle recommendations that can help with your general wellbeing before and during the IVF cycle.

Notes

ACUPUNCTURE

The benefit of Chinese medicine, specifically acupuncture, on fertility is well documented, both in the classics of Chinese medicine and in research carried out worldwide.

Acupuncture is an effective therapy that you can use in preparation for, during and after your IVF cycle. Acupuncture uses tiny, solid needles to stimulate different points in your body that help support various systems. For fertility, acupuncture can be used to not only help with stress but support the body to overcome underlying imbalances that may affect the success of an IVF cycle. Acupuncture also supports and encourages egg health, healthy uterine circulation and lining, hormonal balance, stress impact and much more.

A 2012 meta-analysis found that acupuncture during IVF significantly increases clinical pregnancy rates and live birth rates. The effect is more significant if acupuncture is administered during the ovarian stimulation phase (follicular phase) and not just at embryo transfer.[33]

Acupuncture during ovarian stimulation may help to increase the number of retrieved eggs[34] and increase endometrial thickness.[35] [36] [37]

A recently published randomised controlled trial showed that patients who received acupuncture treatment during the stimulation

[33] Zheng Ch, Huang Gy, Zhang MM et al. Effects of acupuncture on pregnancy rates in women undergoing in vitro fertilization: a systematic review and meta-analysis. Fertil Steril 2012; 97: 599-611.

[34] Isoyama Manca di Villahermosa D, Dos Santos L, Nogueira MB, et al. Influences of acupuncture on the outcomes of in vitro fertilization has failed; a prospective randomised controlled clinical trial. Acupunct Med 2013; 31: 157-61.

[35] Yu W, Horn B, Acacio B, et al. A pilot study evaluating the combination of acupuncture with sildenfil on endometrial thickness. Fertil Steril 2007; 87:23

[36] Ho M, Huang LC, Chang YY, et al. Electro acupuncture reduces uterine artery blood flow impedance in infertile women. Taiwan J Obstet Gynecol 2009; 48: 148-151.

[37] Stener-Victorin E, Waldenstrom U, Andersson SA, et al. Reduction of blood flow impedance in the uterine arteries of infertile women with electro-acupuncture. Hum Reprod 1996; 11: 1314-7.

phase of an IVF cycle had a significantly thicker endometrial lining compared to the control and sham groups (10.3mm vs. 8.7mm vs. 8.5mm, respectively). They also had a statistically greater number of retrieved eggs (8 vs. 6 vs. 6, respectively).[38]

When to begin acupuncture

When using acupuncture in conjunction with IVF, you will want to begin seeing your acupuncturist at least three months before your IVF cycle begins. Find an acupuncturist who specialises in infertility and IVF support since they will have a deep understanding of IVF, can read your hormone blood tests for an understanding of your situation, and can support you during critical times such as egg retrieval, embryo transfer and directly post-transfer.

It is a good idea to provide your acupuncturist with a copy of your IVF treatment protocol so he/she can more accurately plan your acupuncture treatment.

To get the greatest benefit from acupuncture in conjunction with IVF, four stages of treatment are recommended.

Acupuncture for the preconception phase

When undergoing acupuncture during the preparation or preconception phase, the emphasis is on regulating the menstrual cycle (if required), improving ovarian function, egg quality, uterine thickness and sperm quality (if the male partner is being treated as well).

Acupuncture for the follicular/stimulation phase

Acupuncture for the follicular/stimulation (FSH injections) phase is where the body is supported through the actual process of the IVF

[38] Isoyama Manca di Villahermosa D, Dos Santos L, Nogueira MB, et al. Influences of acupuncture on the outcomes of in vitro fertilization has failed; a prospective randomised controlled clinical trial. Acupunct Med 2013; 31: 157-61.

treatment, focusing on supporting the body and egg growth. Point selection varies according to the stage of treatment e.g. it changes with down-regulation or stimulation. As one of the major risks for IVF is poor uterine receptivity at the time of embryo transfer, treatment to increase the thickness and blood supply of the endometrial lining are ideally included in all treatments.

Your acupuncturist should regularly evaluate your response to IVF. He/she may request copies of oestrogen level results, ultrasound scans, the number and size of follicles and the thickness and quality of the endometrial lining. Based on the findings, your acupuncture treatment may be modified accordingly.

Acupuncture for the luteal phase

Acupuncture during the luteal phase may help improve fertilisation and clinical pregnancy rates. Acupuncture may also help reduce the risk of miscarriage in patients undergoing IVF/ICSI. In a study of 238 patients undergoing IVF/ICSI, the first trimester miscarriage rate was significantly lower in the group receiving acupuncture compared with a control group who did not receive acupuncture (31.8 per cent and 40 per cent, respectively).[39]

Acupuncture for the embryo transfer phase

Acupuncture provided before and after embryo transfer may help uterine receptivity. Recent research in Germany has suggested that using acupuncture with IVF increased the pregnancy rate to nearly 50 per cent. A 42 per cent clinical pregnancy rate was achieved in the test group compared to 26 per cent in the control group that did not receive acupuncture. The researchers concluded that acupuncture seems to be a useful tool for improving pregnancy rate after IVF.

[39] Khorram NM. Adjuvant acupuncture reduces first trimester pregnancy loss after IVF. Open J Obstet Gynecol 2012; 02:283-6.

The treatment in this study involved giving acupuncture just before and just after embryo transfer. Points were chosen to relax the uterus and improve blood flow. The researchers concluded that acupuncture may also affect the autonomic nervous system involved in the control of muscles and gland, and thus may make the lining of the uterus more receptive to receiving an embryo.[40]

Acupuncture as an adjunctive therapy

An acupuncture regime has been associated with less stress both before and after embryo transfer, and possibly improved pregnancy rates. Lower perceived stress at the time of embryo transfer may play a role in an improved pregnancy rate.[41]

N.B. Although many acupuncturists recommend acupuncture just before and just after embryo transfer to increase uterine receptivity, unless your IVF clinic has an in-house acupuncturist, my acupuncture colleagues don't always recommend it as it can cause unnecessary stress trying to fit in an acupuncture appointment just before the procedure and just after, especially if there is a distance to travel. From clinical experience, they do not think it makes a significant difference, especially if the patient has been having regular acupuncture treatments.

Other studies supporting acupuncture and IVF

In a randomised clinical trial involving 43 patients undergoing IVF, four weekly acupuncture treatments were found to lead to significantly lower anxiety levels, as compared to no treatment. Acupuncture points used were HT-7, PC-6, CV-17, GV-20.

[40] Paulus WE, Zhang M, Strehler E, El-Danasouri I, Sterzik K (2000). Influence of acupuncture on the pregnancy rate in patients who undergo assisted reproduction therapy, Fertility and Sterility, Vol 77, No 4.

[41] Balk J et. Al. The relationship between perceived stress, acupuncture, and pregnancy rates among IVF patients; a pilot study. Complimentary Ther. Clin Pract. 2010 Aug; 16(3):154-7.

These results suggest that acupuncture may be a beneficial treatment for women undergoing IVF.[42]

In a prospective cohort clinical study involving 67 reproductive-age women experiencing infertility and undergoing IVF, treatment with acupuncture was found to be associated with significant increases in serum cortisol and prolactin - a beneficial effect promoting greater fertility. These results suggest that acupuncture treatment may benefit women undergoing IVF.[43]

[42] Isoyama D, Cordts EB, et al, Acupunct Med, 2012 April 12; [Epub ahead of print]. (Address: Serviço de Reprodução Humana, Faculdade de Medicina do ABC, Santo André, Brazil).

[43] "Changes in serum cortisol and prolactin associated with acupuncture during controlled ovarian hyperstimulation in women undergoing in vitro fertilization-embryo transfer treatment," Magarelli PC, Cridennda DK, et al, Fertil Steril, 2009; 92(6): 1870-9.

Notes

FERTILITY MASSAGE

Massage, particularly Mizan Therapy, is a beneficial therapy that can help you prepare for your IVF procedure. While traditional massage can reduce stress and increase circulation, fertility massage specifically helps to increase circulation to the reproductive system and supports a healthy ovarian-uterine environment.

Fertility massage helps you prepare for your IVF treatment by:

- Increasing circulation to the ovaries and uterus
- Helping reduce stress
- Bringing fresh oxygenated blood to the uterus and ovaries
- Helping diminish pelvic and abdominal adhesions and scarring in the connective tissue from invasive treatments
- Providing emotional release. This can occur when deep massage is performed over the abdomen, which is referred neurochemically as a 'second brain' - connecting directly to the hippocampus, the emotional centre of the brain. It is an area where people can store a lifetime of negative repressed emotions.

Find a registered, qualified massage therapist specialising in fertility massage. They can also provide 'take-home instructions' on abdominal breathing and instruction on self-massage.

Note: Massage should only be done *before* your IVF treatment. Stop when you commence your IVF cycle as you will become very sensitive in the ovarian area as your follicles and eggs mature and your ovaries become larger in response to the FSH/ovarian stimulating injections. It is also not advisable to have massages after the embryos are transferred.

Osteopathy and chiropractic medicine

Another important factor to consider is structural care in relation to fertility. The tenth nerve and sacrum play an important role in controlling bowel, bladder and reproductive function.

Problems with your skeletal system can have a significant impact on your nervous system and reproductive health. Getting a check-up with either an osteopath or chiropractor can have a considerable impact on your fertility.

MORE LIFESTYLE RECOMMENDATIONS

Apart from diet, supplements, acupuncture and massage, tweaking and modifying your lifestyle can have a positive effect on your overall health as you approach your IVF cycle. Remember, fertility is a whole-body event and regular exercise and adequate sleep can support you throughout your IVF journey.

Exercise

Regular exercise is essential for optimum health, helping to maintain an ideal body weight and supporting the stress response. But you must get the balance right when undergoing IVF. It is not a good idea to sign up for a triathlon or marathon before you embark on an IVF cycle! Rather, incorporate some gentle exercise such as walking or yoga that will benefit but not stress your body.

Regular exercise can help improve your quality of life by:

- Regulating healthy blood sugar levels
- Burning excess body fat and building muscle, in turn boosting your metabolism
- Strengthening your immune system and making you more resistant to illness
- Boosting your stamina and energy
- Lifting your mood and self-confidence
- Reducing the impact of stress on your health
- Improving insulin sensitivity if PCOS is an issue
- Helping lower cholesterol and protecting you from heart disease
- Improving circulation and reducing cellulite.

Ideally, you should enjoy your exercise, especially if it's going to be part of your everyday life. Try to vary it and make it interesting. If you need motivation and encouragement, do it with a friend and have twice as much fun!

Top exercise tips

- Do something every day. This could be walking, swimming, yoga or Pilates.
- Walking is free and you can walk almost anywhere. It is one of the best overall fitness activities; it places very little strain on your joints and involves all the major muscle groups. Walk to work, get off one stop earlier from the train or bus, go for a walk during your lunch break, or take the stairs instead of the lift. Ideally walk where there are hills to increase your heart rate.
- Don't overexert yourself but do make sure you exercise sufficiently to raise your heart rate for at least 20 minutes (enough to raise a sweat) three to five times a week. Reduce exercise if you are unwell.
- If you need extra motivation, you can download exercise program applications onto your smart phone that you can follow.

Exercise for weight loss

The more your body is active, the more fat you will burn and the healthier your whole body will be. Even if you are a healthy weight, exercise is still very important. So, get moving!

Sleep

If you are reading this book in bed with your e-book reader, stop! Turn it off, take it out of the room, along with your mobile phone. If you still want to read in bed, read this book in a paperback version or choose a light-hearted novel to help you relax and go to sleep.

> In December 2014, the National Academy of Science published the findings from researchers at Boston's Brigham and Women's Hospital of a suppressive effect for evening use of light-emitting electronic devices on sleep and melatonin secretion.
>
> Electronic devices emit light that is short-wavelength-enriched light, which has a higher concentration of blue light, with a peak around 450 nm than natural light. This is different from natural light in composition, having a greater impact on sleep and circadian rhythms.
>
> The eBook reading was associated with more time needed to fall asleep and less rapid eye movement sleep in comparison with reading a printed book. Evening melatonin levels were suppressed by an average of 55.12 per cent in eBook readers, while those who read printed books had no suppression. Compared to printed book reading, the onset of melatonin release in response to dim light occurred 1.5 hours later the day following the reading of an eBook.
>
> A more surprising finding was that individuals using the e-reader would be more tired and take longer to become alert the next morning.
>
> We live in a sleep-restricted society. More study is warranted on the effects of using light-emitting devices, especially before bed, as they may have longer-term health consequences than previously considered.

Get adequate sleep

Preparing for sleep the night before is the place to start. The quantity and quality of sleep is vital. A busy mind leading to broken sleep does not allow for a fresh mind on waking.

Why else is sleep so important?

Lots of metabolic processes occur when we sleep. For one, glutathione, a detoxification enzyme, is activated during sleep, so your body is detoxifying while you sleep. Other processes that occur during sleep include blood sugar rebalancing and reduction of stress hormones such as adrenalin and cortisol.

Try some of these simple steps to help you sleep well and wake well.

1. Avoid caffeine.

2. Avoid alcohol.

3. Avoid heavy, rich evening meals as they can lead to digestive discomfort during the night and sluggish feelings in the morning.

4. Sleeping in a cool and dark room allows you to enjoy a more restful sleep.

5. Before you go to bed, write a quick note on any thoughts that are in your brain (such as work stressors). Getting them out allows you to release them until the next day.

6. Get some sleep before midnight. It is said that one hour of sleep before midnight equates to two hours of sleep quality after midnight. Ideally get to bed no later than 10pm if you are due to wake up at 6am.

7. For circulating unwanted thoughts at night, try a few drops of White Chestnut Bach flower drops under your tongue before you go to bed.

8. If you wake and are sluggish, start with a cold shower or a brisk walk around the block, they both bring energy quickly to a tired soul.

9. Roll over and enjoy a moment with your partner, don't just race off to get into the work day. Even if you are busy, take a moment to be with them and make your heart smile.

10. Use essential oils like clary-sage, geranium and chamomile in a vaporiser at bedtime to help you switch off and ground yourself so that you can enjoy quality sleep. These simple and earthy blends stop your mind racing so that you can focus on one thing at a time, like sleeping. They help to restore some peace and balance to your life during the busiest of times. These essential oils are also indicated to help female infertility.

11. You can also vaporise citrus or leaf essential oils like orange, lemongrass or grapefruit in the morning to enliven you and kick-start your day. These essential oils will help lift you physically and emotionally. Regain the feeling that you are really living and not just existing.

12. If you experience problems with insomnia, your naturopath may prescribe nutrients such as 5-HTP (serotonin precursor) and magnesium, plus herbal teas such as Chamomile and Lemon Balm for their relaxing and soothing properties.

Notes

RELATIONSHIP SUPPORT

Infertility issues and IVF can place a huge strain on even the strongest of relationships especially if you don't know what to expect.

It's important to be prepared for a few ups and downs. The combination of continuous medical intervention, high expectations and disappointments can turn IVF into a real emotional rollercoaster for a couple.

The good news is you will likely be offered counselling to help you, and there's a lot you can do as a couple to keep your relationship loving, happy and strong.

Based on my and the collective experience of many IVF couples, here are some tips on reducing the collateral damage on your relationship during your IVF journey.

Share your feelings

The important thing is to share your experiences and remember you're going through this together, not alone.

It is a stereotype, but it is often the men who don't share their feelings as much as women. Of the couples I see in my clinic, it is often the women experiencing the rollercoaster of emotions while the men seem to be the (supposedly) strong, silent ones.

The key to sustaining your relationship during the IVF journey is to resolve the small things that happen in your life and try not to think about the 'what ifs' that lie ahead. Try not to assume what the other is thinking as this can lead to unnecessary misunderstandings and possible arguments. Rather, spend time talking and sharing your thoughts. Being able to communicate is vital. Talk about how best you can support each other, working as a team for the IVF journey.

The difference between men and women

Although men want a baby too, the desire a woman has to have a baby is not always as strongly felt by a man.

Women can be much more emotionally sensitive during an IVF cycle, especially if there have been unsuccessful cycles previously. It is not uncommon for women to become more teary and cry.

It is also not unusual for sex to be on the backburner during the IVF journey. Women especially can find it difficult to feel intimate or have sex when they are coping with a barrage of emotions such as feelings of uncertainty, disappointment, anger, resentment or even grief.

Men want to provide a solution (thanks to their logical reasoning) but sadly they cannot always offer this. The best thing a man can do is hold his partner, sympathise with her and try to encourage her to look forward with hope.

At the same time, it is important to respect that men and women experience and deal with emotions differently. Usually women want to talk, whereas men generally need a bit of time and space on their own to think and reflect.

It is good for men to share how they feel about the IVF journey with their partner but allow them space and the right time to talk.

Here are some relationship-strengthening tips:

- Take time out together – go away for a weekend, go for a walk or picnic, catch a movie, anything that gives you a breather from the intensity of IVF.
- Set aside time to talk when you know you will not be interrupted – away from distractions such as television and social media.

- Listen to each other and try not to blame each other for the way you are feeling. Express how you are feeling and how a situation has made you feel.
- Don't say things you will regret in the heat of the moment. This can often happen during an argument.

IVF counselling

Sadly, sometimes going through IVF can bring out the worst in a couple. For others, it can bring them closer together. Men tend to be more logical and women tend to be more emotional, but essentially, we all want the same things out of a relationship – to feel connected, loved, understood and in harmony with each other emotionally. If you are struggling, seek professional help sooner rather than later. Most IVF clinics offer counselling.

IVF/fertility counselling can help couples to resolve conflicts related to the pressures of infertility and the actual process of an IVF cycle. It is important that you are both able to talk about your feelings and concerns. Simply acknowledging some of these concerns goes a long way to resolving them and finding a middle ground where necessary.

Lastly, remember to have some fun in your relationship. Remember to laugh out loud. Build on your strengths and support one another.

Notes

FLOWER ESSENCES

Flower essences are gentle in action yet can provide profound shifts on a mental, emotional and energetic level.

The original Bach Flower Remedies were developed in the 1930s by Dr Edward Bach, a well-known Harley Street doctor and homoeopath. He viewed illness as the result of conflict between body and mind, with symptoms being the external expression of negative emotional states. This internal war, according to Bach, causes a lack of harmony in the body, blocking energy and leading to physical diseases.

Since then, other flower essences have been identified worldwide.

Flower essences can profoundly support women through the emotional ups and downs of the IVF journey. They help put us more in control of our feelings. There are Bach flower remedies, Australian Bush Flower essences and Bailey flower essences, among others. They are equally useful to men and women to help gain back inner balance at the mental and emotional level during times of stress and anxiety. They can be taken during fertility treatment such as IVF (and even during pregnancy) as they are non-toxic, act gently and don't have side effects.

> *"Bach remedies are beneficent in action, and cause no aggravation nor reaction, for their effect is to uplift."*
>
> Dr Edward Bach, 1930

Bach Flower Remedies

The following are examples of Bach Flower Remedies.

Agrimony – a remedy for inner anguish, when you hide your feeling by putting on a brave face and don't show others your true worrying feelings about getting pregnant.

Gentian – a great remedy for setbacks, disappointments and feeling discouraged such as when an IVF cycle has failed. It helps to lift your spirit to optimism.

Impatience - If you feel impatient and irritable about not getting pregnant fast enough, Impatiens helps eliminate that feeling of nervous anticipation, promoting serenity and helping you relax a little more while you wait. Impatiens helps you stay calm during the two-week wait after embryo transfer.

Mimulus – a remedy for specific fears and for those who are very shy and fearful. This remedy will be helpful if you are fearful of any parts of the IVF procedure, including injections, blood tests and egg retrieval.

Olive – for mental and physical fatigue. Olive also helps give you energy during the IVF process.

Pine – for feelings of guilt and self-blame. Pine helps release your sense of guilt no matter what the cause. This negative emotion can create emotional blocks that can hamper treatment success.

White Chestnut – a great remedy for persistent worrying thoughts, especially at night when you find yourself constantly thinking and worrying about possible outcomes. White Chestnut helps you deal with these unwanted thoughts, clearing your mind and promoting relaxation.

Australian Bush Flower Essences

The Australian Bush Flower Essences by Ian White work in a similar way to the Bach Flower Remedies but come from different flower essences commonly found in Australia. Many naturopaths find these more suitable for 'modern day' problems and very powerful.

Flannel Flower Essence – 'you've lost that loving feeling...', a great remedy for couples who are so worried about the outcome and cannot focus on enjoying their time together as a couple. It is said to bring enjoyment through physical contact like touching and feeling once more.

She Oak Flower Essence – if there is one essence you should have, if you are struggling with fertility issues, it is She Oak! This essence is very beneficial for hormone imbalances and bringing about a sense of wellbeing. A great remedy for those who feel distressed about their infertility. It can also help you release any emotional blocks associated with negative feeling, which might inhibit conception at the emotional level.

Turkey Bush Flower Essence – a useful essence while trying to conceive because creativity and conception are at the same soul level. If you experience discouragement as a result of not being able to 'create a new life', these negative emotions can create emotional blocks that can be cleared by Turkey Bush.

Australian Bush Flower Blends

Emergency Essence – The Australian version of Bach's Rescue Remedy, this combination is excellent for acute stress and worry after an accident or shock. It can be taken throughout the IVF journey – from the injections stage and egg retrieval to embryo transfer and during the two-week wait after embryo transfer. This is a great combination to take when getting over the disappointment of implantation failure or a 'BFN' (Big Fat Negative').

Purifying Essence - this is a powerfully cleansing essence on both a physical and emotional level. This blend of essences contains Dagger Hakea, which helps with forgiveness. Bottlebrush, as the name describes, is like a brush cleaning out the old emotional baggage we no longer need while clearing the bowel on a physical level. Wild Potato Bush may help clear toxins from the body and is great for renewing enthusiasm. Bauhinia helps when a person resists change or holds on to negative emotions. This blend can help purify your physical and emotional body, so you are ready for your forthcoming IVF cycle, potential pregnancy and baby.

Relationship Essence – a good choice if you feel your relationship is under stress or requires nurturing. If there is any built-up resentment or problems in the relationship, this essence is indicated to soften and restore communication before restoring sexual intimacy.

Woman Essence - contains the flower essence She Oak, which supports the female reproductive system (ovaries, uterus) and harmonises these organs. Bush Fuchsia helps support the hypothalamus and pituitary glands, which can affect ovulation. The essence Old Man Banksia supports the thyroid function and Five Corners is especially useful for self-esteem. This is a fantastic pre-conception tonic, bringing a woman into her feminine power - a great blend to use throughout an IVF cycle, pregnancy, birth and beyond.

Bailey Flower Essences

Bailey essences are primarily concerned with personal growth and liberation. This does not mean that the essences cannot help physical illnesses – far from it. Yet their main emphasis is on helping integrate mind, body and spirit. These flower essences help us to open our eyes and see things as they really are; to let go of fears and to discover the real power that lies at the heart of each one of us; to discover more about ourselves than perhaps we ever dreamt possible.

Like the other flower essences, they are not drugs so they do not force change, but they will help us to change if we are ready for change to take place. They are therefore gentle but persuasive in their action.

Apricot Poppy - brings beauty to barren areas of our lives. Its soft, quiet persistence is what we need to survive upheaval and trauma. It opens the door so that we may access the unlearned wisdom of the intuitive mind. It gently beckons us forward, away from stagnation. It whispers to us the messages that we need to hear and encourages us to keep going forwards in our life, embracing change and knowledge with joy rather than dread.

Arizona Fir - the essence of Arizona Fir is about celebrating life and existence. Clinging to our current path of suffering is disastrous to our personal well-being, and it closes doors to other possibilities. It is the clinging that is the problem. We need to open up and rejoice in life, to love life, to love our own selves. Arizona Fir softens our rigidity and opens the door to the mysteries of true celebration.

Bladder Senna - helps free us from guilt from the past. Guilt is very destructive. We need to escape the tyranny of severe self-judgement and accept that we occasionally get things wrong. It is a flower of self-compassion and understanding.

Buttercup - for those who need to open up and let the sunshine into their lives. They may have been badly treated in the past and their confidence in others has been severely shaken. They may have become quite cutting and cynical as a result.

Compact Rush - for those who feel that life is passing them by. They dwell on opportunities that had denied them. This sadness is suppressed anger that things were not different. They feel disempowered and resentful. Compact Rush is about new beginnings, fresh starts, a clean slate. Embrace the present moment with new energies and new insight.

Dog Rose - for help and loving comfort and support when life gets difficult. The hurt may have gone deep where no-one can reach and help. Dog Rose gives relief from this feeling, and helps our heart to protect itself, developing our loving and compassionate nature.

Fuji Cherry - helps us relax and take life less seriously. The key essence for developing a calm and quiet mind. There is a close link between mind and body tensions.

Holly Leaf - helps us see things as they really are and therefore to let go of pent-up anger and bitterness. It is a protective essence so that we do not become angry so easily.

Honeysuckle - sadness and loneliness isolate us from other people. Honeysuckle brings ease and comfort to our hearts and pulls down over-protective barriers that we may have erected between ourselves and the world around us. It also carries our own beautiful fragrances out to the world to attract love and healing towards ourselves.

Ivy - simply keeps our feet on the ground. It roots us in the physical world where we can feel secure and loved. A great essence for grounding as well as for shock.

Lily of the Valley – a remedy for yearning. For those who have become blocked by desiring the unattainable. Behind the yearning there is a sense of desperation and of being incomplete until the desire is achieved. Paradoxically, the answer lies in giving up the search. Lily of the Valley helps create 'the empty cup' so that what we truly need can find the space within us and enter in. It is an essence of trust.

Scabious - for healing us when we need gentleness and quiet support. It helps us see that even serious problems may have very positive outcomes that we cannot possibly envisage at the time.

Sheep's Sorrel - for feelings of bitterness when we feel that life is desperately unfair.

White Cherry - from time to time we find ourselves in the grip of some emotion that has its roots in the distant past. White Cherry helps to dissipate negative influences, dissolving old cellular memories. This is a very powerful healing and cleansing essence.

White Lotus - peace and tranquillity at all levels of the consciousness. It's a great aid in meditation to quiet the chattering mind. It mirrors our sitting in quiet wonderment at the true beauty of everything in this astonishing universe. Attitudes and opinions fall away leaving only pure awareness.

Yorkshire Fog - encourages unshed tears to fall. Trapped grief is harmful to body and soul. Tears are a natural way to wash away anger, frustration and sadness. Accepting our hurt and anguish is a necessary part of the healing process. Yorkshire Fog helps us move on after the tears to a new and changed future.

How to make flower essences

Flower essences can be taken with other medicines and alongside other naturopathic and homoeopathic remedies, including supplements.

Your naturopath may select the most suitable remedies for you or you may self-select based on your mental and emotional state.

The best method is to make a prescription bottle. A prescription bottle is a 30ml amber bottle that can be purchased from a pharmacy or provided by your naturopath. Fill the bottle with 30ml of spring water (or 50 per cent vodka and 50 per cent water for longer-keeping properties) and each essence selected. In the case of alcohol intolerance, salt can be used. In this case, add approximately 25 per cent by weight of sea-salt to the spring water and shake it until all the salt has dissolved.

Essence	Bach Flower Remedies	Australian Bush Essences	Bailey Flower Essences
Prescription bottle	2 drops	7 drops	2 drops
Dose	4 drops 4 times daily under your tongue	7 drops twice daily under your tongue	3 drops three times daily under your tongue

If the problems are acute, then the prescription can be taken more frequently – every hour or so if needed. This is most likely where sudden shock has occurred, for example, where there has been a 'BFN', implantation failure or miscarriage.

If no dropper bottles are available, then the drops of each of the selected essences can be added to a small glass of water. A small amount of this can then be sipped two to four times per day depending on the essence. If it is kept refrigerated, this mixture has a useful life of about three days, after which a new mixture will need to be prepared.

Normally it is best for the whole bottle to be taken. However, if symptoms are changing rapidly, it may be advisable to check more frequently – say, every week – and adjust the prescription to reflect your changing needs.

Up to five essences can be given at any one time. More than this is not normally recommended. Here it should be noted that the composite (blends) essences can be treated in exactly the same way as a single essence. If more than five appear to be needed, then it may be better to split the essences into two separate prescriptions. These could then be taken in alternate weeks, or the two prescriptions could be alternated day by day. Be guided by your naturopath as to which course of action to take.

BIORESONANCE THERAPY

Infertility issues may also be assisted with bioresonance therapy, a non-invasive, gentle therapy that uses biophysics - the physics of your body to reduce your toxin and stress load, clear pathogenic loads such as Epstein Barr virus, Chlamydia bacterial and other microorganism infections, balance your hormone levels and restore your body's ability to heal itself.

Bioresonance is based on the scientific principle that metabolism within cells is influenced by one's own electromagnetic field. There are no harmful side effects.

The therapy uses electromagnetic waves and frequency patterns with machines such as the German state-of-the-art BICOM machine. It identifies normal healthy cells and unhealthy viruses, bacteria, allergens and toxins. It then strengthens the healthy waves to increase normal functions and inverts unhealthy waves with an electronic mirror circuit to cancel out the harmful waves that are stressing your body.

The process is obviously a lot more complicated and the number of therapy sessions may depend on the complexity of symptoms.

Bioresonance technology can be used for both female and male infertility issues and is recommended during the preconception period.

Notes

Section 7

Surviving the two-week wait

During the two-week wait after embryo transfer, you can be on an emotional rollercoaster ride, from experiencing sheer excitement to fluctuating levels of anxiety, made worse by the thought of possible IVF failure.

Even in cases where all has gone seemingly well, you may still feel anxious during this phase.

The two-week wait is a quieter period of time of the IVF process. You go from having regular scans and blood tests, egg retrieval, and embryo transfer to almost nothing while awaiting D-day, pregnancy test day! This is a time where emotional support is very important.

I know it is tempting to jump onto every IVF forum and read what might be happening to others every day of the two-week wait, and to research any little niggling feelings you may have, but please don't!

It is easier said than done, I know. In the early days of my first few IVF cycles, I did it myself. But on subsequent cycles, I dedicated time to practising the breathing, meditation and visualisation techniques detailed in this book.

It is important to try to let go of the stress, tension, worry and anguish. Relaxation techniques such as visualisation and meditation have been shown to help release feel-good endorphins and increase blood flow to the reproductive organs, including the uterus.

Total relaxation is a skill you need to practise and learn. Practising a relaxation technique even just 20 minutes a day will help you experience deep relaxation and maintain a calm, yet positive mind and attitude.

Lastly, spend time with nurturing and uplifting friends and family members. Take time out and go for a walk, amble around some markets or see a movie. Surround yourself with those who love and support you.

BREATHING EXERCISES

Hi Lo Breathing is a wonderful relaxing breathing technique that can be practised several times daily.

You can practise this breathing technique lying down for better effect; however, it can be practised in a seated position once you are familiar with it.

Place one hand on your chest, one hand on your abdomen, breath in through your nose and out through your mouth, exhaling as if gently blowing through a straw.

Listen to your breathing and note which hand is moving most, try and take your breathing down to your abdomen with very little movement from your upper hand. This should feel natural to you and without strain.

When you are comfortable with the above, start your breathing, inhaling for a count of four and exhaling for a count of four. Think about mobilising your rib cage and enhancing your breathing muscles. This means breathing wide and full into the side and back of your ribs, feeling your ribs open up like an umbrella on the inhalation, and letting them soften and close down on the exhalation. At the same time, feel yourself lift up from your diaphragm (easier if you are in the seated position).

Practise this breathing technique twice daily for a few minutes, on waking, bedtime and before meals. You can practise every hour if you are feeling anxious or stressed.

When this breathing technique feels natural to you, perhaps after a week, start to lengthen your breaths by varying the counts e.g. inhale for three counts and exhale for five. Then try inhaling for four counts and exhaling for six.

Don't rush to change your breathing pattern - it is supposed to be a nice, slow process.

Notes

MEDITATION

Meditation involves relieving the thinking mind by placing yourself into a deep state of awareness and relaxation. It may be practised sitting up or lying down and is best done somewhere private and quiet where you won't be disturbed for at least 5–20 minutes (or longer) at a time.

Meditation techniques

While there are hundreds of meditation techniques available, all fit into one of the following categories:

- Concentration meditation, where the mind is focused on a specific object. When the mind wanders into old thought patterns, you bring your focus back to the object.
- Mindfulness meditation, where the mind is focused on an object or your breath, a mantra or a visual image.
- Transcendental meditation, in which you experience a shift in consciousness or physiology.

The benefits of meditating

Meditation works to relieve symptoms of stress by helping you relax. This improves your stress response.

Meditation:

- Slows down the breath and helps you breathe more efficiently
- Increases vital blood supply to the reproductive organs including the uterus
- Normalises blood pressure and decreases your heart rate
- Reduces cortisol (the 'stress' hormone) production from the adrenal glands
- Improves glucose metabolism

- Reduces inflammation
- Regulates the appetite
- Reduces the rate of ageing
- Improves overall immunity levels
- Increases self-awareness
- Reduces negative emotions
- Gives new perspective on stressful situations
- Guides you to focus on the present moment.

VISUALISATION

Regardless of whether you have been on the fertility rollercoaster for a while, or have had repeated unsuccessful IVF cycles, visualisation can be very powerful. Don't underestimate the power of the mind. I recommend visualisation to help women replace negative self-sabotaging thoughts with positive thoughts and to reconnect with their bodies.

Being able to visualise or see pictures or images through techniques that incorporate breathing, meditation or listening to a CD can help you relax and keep you positive. My *'Guided Meditation for IVF Success'* CD will support you through your fertility and IVF journey.

Below is a beautiful visualisation technique adapted from the wonderful Ishayas meditation group.
www.thebrightpath.com

Guided Pink Light visualisation

The following visualisation technique is a powerful healing tool that may be practised daily. This technique has been used for centuries for healing purposes.

1. Get yourself in a comfortable position. This may be lying down or seated. Now, remember a time when you felt loved.

2. In your mind's eye, picture Pink Loving Light radiating from your heart, encompassing you in a Pink Sphere.

3. Stay within your Pink Light Sphere - remember a loving memory of yourself (this could be recent or from your childhood) and project this aspect of you outside of the Pink Light Sphere. Cover this projection of yourself with the Pink Loving Light (radiating from your heart).

4. Then, starting with your immediate family - mother, father, siblings, partner, children - individually imagine them in front of you, outside the Pink Light Sphere. If possible, have the image of them in a loving memory. In your mind's eye, picture yourself covering each of them with the Pink Light (as if you were icing a cake). Cover them, and then let them go and move on to the next person. (If you cannot remember this person in a loving memory, just picture them in front of you. If you cannot do this, then bring them in, standing at a distance and/or facing away from you).

5. Now imagine the tiny beautiful embryo(s) that are either waiting to be transferred, have been frozen or have already been transferred to your warm, nourishing and nurturing womb. Cover them with the Pink Light, imagining them growing and implanting into the lining of your womb.

6. Next, bring in anyone with whom you still have an emotional charge or discomfort. (Follow the instructions above).

7. Allow for anyone else to show up (whoever needs to be brought into your awareness is OK), cover them with the Pink Loving Light and let them go as well.

Note: In the beginning, this process should take no more than ten minutes a day, eventually getting down to five minutes. If you can't visualise the Pink Light, that is fine, the intent is what is important.

Practise this daily during the two-week wait. Cover your embryo(s) with the Pink Loving Light. Most importantly, remember to bathe yourself in the healing Pink Light.

You can follow this guided pink light visualisation on my audio *'Guided Meditation for IVF Success'*. Available for download from ivfdiet.com

Section 8

When IVF doesn't work

Sadly not all IVF cycles will be successful.

When you find out that the cycle hasn't worked, it is devastating. There are so many 'whys' and 'what did I do wrong' and 'what could I have done differently' questions.

But it is important to not blame yourself or anyone else. Sometimes doctors may have an inkling where things have gone wrong, but otherwise, sadly and frustratingly, there may be no answers.

These days, pregnancy tests are so much more sensitive than generations ago, so a test can show positive very early on when the embryo is making its first tentative attempts at implantation. Essentially the diagnosis of pregnancy is made based on identifying human chorionic gonadotropin hormone (better known as HCG), which is getting earlier and earlier. Physiologically there may be little difference between an embryo not implanting at a matter of a few days or a few weeks, but once a pregnancy test has shown positive, quite understandably this tends to take on a whole other meaning for a woman when she then miscarriages.

The pain of miscarriage

Many doctors believe there is a crossover between implantation failure in IVF and recurrent miscarriage. Implantation can be thought as a continuous process starting at the time the blastocyst starts to implant in the endometrium (uterine lining) and completing by around 12 weeks of pregnancy when the placenta takes over the full hormonal production.

While modern technology is very good at making embryos in the laboratory, doctors still cannot control the implantation process. They do not know which embryo will become a baby - and this can be very frustrating, for both patients and doctors. How implantation is regulated and brought about remains an enigma, but we need to remember that the implantation process is surprisingly inefficient in humans - nature is not always very competent. Embryo implantation is a complex process, so there is no need to blame yourself if the embryos do not implant.

Many of the reasons why a woman has recurrent miscarriages are the same as for women who have recurrent implantation failure at IVF.

These can include:

- Age
- Genetic factors within the embryo (most common reason)
- Abnormal chromosomes in women and men
- Hormonal imbalances (including elevated prolactin and PCOS)
- Low progesterone levels
- Blood clotting disorders
- Immune disorders
- Infections such as Parvo virus, ureaplasma, mycoplasma, Listeria and Strep B
- Structural abnormalities of the uterus (womb) and cervix
- Obesity and subsequent complications
- Lifestyle factors – poor diet, caffeine, smoking, alcohol, drugs, radiation and toxic exposure.

Having a miscarriage is a highly emotional experience for a woman, as well as being a shocking and painful physical experience and a more subtle hormonal one. I remember my own experience of miscarriage.

It doesn't ease the pain to learn that half of all pregnancies end in miscarriage. Nor to be told that one can always try again.

Investigating miscarriage

In the UK, the cause of miscarriage isn't investigated until it occurs for a third time, which can be very difficult for women. We know enough to recognise there are factors in a family or in a woman's history that might make her more prone to miscarriage.

Investigations for recurrent miscarriage usually start with a blood test to see if there are any hormonal imbalances. The blood clotting factors will be checked, chromosomes tested for both the woman and her partner, and a full infection screened performed.

Sometimes there may be no physical signs of a miscarriage such as bleeding or cramps, and the first indication of a problem may be at a scan to confirm everything is going well. To be told at that stage that there is no heartbeat, or the pregnancy is not progressing as it should is devastating – creating anger, disbelief and enormous sadness.

Some women will miscarry naturally but at other times the miscarriage may be incomplete, and an operation is required usually under general anaesthetic. This is known as an ERPCI - evacuation of retained products of conception. Some people still refer to this procedure as a D&C (dilation and curettage). There are many medical ways to manage miscarriage, which involve the use of pills and pessaries, but the management of miscarriage will depend on many factors.

Women who have undergone IVF to conceive and then miscarry in the first trimester experience more stress and emotional trauma for at least three months afterwards than women who have conceived naturally and who then miscarry.[44]

Clearly miscarriage is a huge topic and a book such as this cannot possibly do it justice.

[44] Cheung C, Chan C, Ng E. Stress and anxiety-depression levels following first-trimester miscarriage: a comparison between women who conceived naturally and women who conceived with assisted reproduction. NJOG 2013; 120: 1090-7.

DEALING WITH IMPLANTATION FAILURE OR A MISCARRIAGE

Women (and men) can experience such extreme high and low emotions during the IVF journey that it can really take a toll on their overall health and wellbeing.

It is important to come to terms with the emotions you experience after an implantation failure or miscarriage so that anxiety doesn't affect your next attempt at IVF, because as we know, anxiety is in itself a stressor to the body.

What you must do is to be positive. The good news is some of the reasons why it doesn't work are modifiable. You can lose weight, reduce toxin exposure, eat a healthier diet and take supplements to improve your health. You can avoid caffeine and stop smoking and drinking. You can be supported mentally and emotionally.

Look at all these aspects of your health and lifestyle and review both the **Preconception Preparation Plan** outlined in Section 2, the **IVF Diet Guidelines** in Section 4, and the *IVF Support Guide for Men* to give you and your partner the best chance of a successful pregnancy.

Naturopathic support

For many couples who have experienced a miscarriage, becoming pregnant can bring on the worry that miscarriage could happen again. For those who have endured recurrent miscarriages, pregnancy is a time of fear and trepidation, and any slight twinge can induce an emotional rollercoaster.

The best time for a woman with a history of implantation failure or miscarriage to see a naturopath is long before conception is attempted. As mentioned in the Preconception section, if time permits, it is best to have at least three months of treatment in advance of an IVF cycle. A naturopathic approach takes time because the body needs time to heal and change. Three months is considered the minimum, since each new follicle and each new sperm has a journey of approximately three months until maturity.

The treatments that are typically considered are nutrition (diet and supplements), herbal medicine, homoeopathy, acupuncture, aromatherapy, flower essences, physical therapies and counselling. Your naturopath may consider one or more of these treatments and may also include other treatments not mentioned in this chapter. You may also consider seeing a practitioner who is focused in one particular area of treatment, such as a homoeopath or acupuncturist. Whatever route you choose, it is important that you have a therapist who is sensitive to the issue of IVF implantation failure and miscarriage and comfortable discussing the physical and emotional concerns that may arise.

Diet

As outlined in this book, a healthy diet consisting of an abundance of fruits, vegetables, whole rains, healthy fats and quality protein is recommended. Depending on your history, you may also be advised to avoid dairy products or gluten, or both. There could be a number of reasons for this, but a primary concern is the health of the immune system and its possible implication in recurrent miscarriage.

It is also wise to avoid any foods that may harbour the bacteria Listeria as it can lead to miscarriage or stillbirth. High-risk foods that often contain Listeria are cold foods such as paté, deli meats, pre-mixed salads, soft-serve ice-cream, soft cheeses, smoked seafood and any leftovers kept in the refrigerator for more than 12 hours.

Nutritional supplements

Your naturopath may prescribe specific supplements to assist in the prevention of miscarriage, particularly if a cause has been identified.

Some examples include active folate (5-methyltetrahydrofolate), Coenzyme Q10, DHEA and vitamin E.

Note: It is important to not self-prescribe but be advised by your naturopath and/or doctor.

For more information, please refer to Section 5, Supplements.

Herbal medicine

There are some effective herbs that are used to help prevent miscarriage. You may be prescribed a liquid extract blend or tincture containing herbs such as False Unicorn Root, Black Cohosh, Motherwort and Peony which can be taken in the preconception months or in the case of False Unicorn Root, after embryo transfer.

It is imperative that you take all of these herbs under the guidance of your naturopath or herbalist. If you are beginning IVF treatment, it is important that you stop taking all forms of herbal medicine as soon as you begin your fertility drugs, unless otherwise prescribed.

For more information, please refer to Section 5, Herbal Medicines.

Homoeopathy

The word homoeopathy comes from the Greek words, *homos* (meaning 'same') and *pathos* (meaning 'suffering'). In homoeopathy, different people suffering from the same problem can be given different remedies because each person is treated according to their individual symptoms and constitution. Because infertility and miscarriage is multi-factorial, it is better to consult a qualified homoeopath so that the treatment is individualised.

Homoeopathic medicine has been safely prescribed for over 200 years and is a respected and widely used therapy. It is estimated that the majority of European homoeopathic practitioners are also medical doctors.

Homoeopathy is a modality of healing similar to acupuncture. It induces energetic shifts, and because of this energetic approach to treatment, is completely safe to use even during pregnancy. (Please note: homoeopathy is not herbal medicine.) Homoeopathic remedies, when carefully chosen, can help prevent future miscarriage, and are successful in roughly 70 per cent of threatened miscarriage cases. It is important to acknowledge that homoeopathy will not prevent miscarriage if the pregnancy is not viable. In those cases, homoeopathic medicine can be used to ease the woman's discomfort and calm her.

There are many homoeopathic remedies that may be prescribed. It is always best to consult with an experienced practitioner and to not self-prescribe. In general, though, there is one homoeopathic remedy, Sabina, in a potency of 6c, 12c or 30c, that can be taken as a preventative once per week for the first 20 weeks of pregnancy, and also every four hours in case of a threatened miscarriage. However, keep in mind that this is a general recommendation, and may not be the best approach for everyone.

Other commonly used homoeopathic remedies that may be prescribed include Arnica, Caulophyllum, Cimicifuga, Kali carb, Crocus sativa, Erigeron, Helonias, Secale, Sepia and Ustilago, among constitutional remedies. Regarding Arnica, if given on time, it can, in rare cases, remove the threatened miscarriage.

Acupuncture

Acupuncture can be very effective in helping prevent miscarriage in some instances. It can also be highly effective for threatened miscarriage. By nourishing a woman's reproductive organs, healing and balance can be restored after a miscarriage.

However, as with homoeopathy, if the pregnancy is not viable, then the acupuncture will not prevent pregnancy loss.

Aromatherapy

The essential oils recommended for use after implantation failure or miscarriage assist in healing on the physical, mental and emotional level. Choose a single oil or make yourself a blend using the oils below, adding 1 drop of essential oil to each millilitre of base oil for a body oil and 6-8 drops in a bath:

- Frankincense - 9 drops
- Geranium - 5 drops
- Grapefruit - 7 drops
- Chamomile Roman - 9 drops.

Flower essences

Emotions around an IVF failure or miscarriage range from grief, disappointment and guilt. No matter which part of our pregnancy we lose a baby, it is devastating. Flower essences can assist with the emotions that miscarriage brings.

Bach Flower Remedies may include:

- Cherry Plum: helps us when we are on the verge of breakdown; and when we are in deep despair and feel that we are going to lose our sanity. Cherry Plum helps us to be calm and think and act rationally.
- Gorse: helps us when we feel extreme hopelessness and despair. Gorse gives us a sense of faith and hope.
- Pine: helps us when we feel guilt for failure or loss. Pine helps us be realistic and not blame ourselves unnecessarily.
- Star of Bethlehem: helps us deal with the trauma, devastation and disappointment of losing a baby at any stage of pregnancy. It helps neutralise the effect of the trauma and aids in recuperation.
- Sweet Chestnut: helps us when we feel that we have reached the limit of our endurance and the future is hopeless. Sweet Chestnut helps us regain optimism and faith in a higher power and gives us a sense of inner support.

- Willow: helps us when we feel the grief has turned into resentment and self-pity. Willow helps us regain faith and optimism and we will once more be able to enjoy life.

The Australian Bush Flower essence blend 'Emergency Essence' and the Bailey Flower essence blend 'Shock and Trauma' are both also excellent for any panic, distress, fear and emotional upset. They have a calming effect during a crisis and assists in the ability to cope. They encourage comfort and reassurance. Administer these remedies every hour or more frequently if necessary, until you feel better.

Refer to Section 6 for more information on flower essences.

Physical therapies

Massage is an excellent physical therapy to consider helping improve uterine circulation, and so, like acupuncture, can be an effective way to prevent miscarriage.

Refer to Section 6 for more information on massage.

Castor oil packs can ease pain and discomfort. It involves applying the castor oil pack to the abdomen, with either a hot water bottle or heating pad placed on top for warmth. The pack should remain in place for at least 30 minutes. Castor oil packs increase circulation and lymphatic activity; they have also been observed to dissolve scar tissue. However, they should be used only during the first half of the cycle, and **not** when you are pregnant.

For instruction on creating Castor Oil packs, please refer to my website, jennyblondel.com.

In summary

For women who are struggling with their fertility, implantation failure or a miscarriage is not just a little bump along the road of her life; it can be a significant setback. It can take time to heal. Be kind to yourself.

I hope by reading this you feel reassured that there are natural, holistic therapies that can assist in the healing and recovery after an implantation failure or miscarriage.

Notes

Section 9

When IVF works

First and foremost, congratulations if you have been successful with IVF and are finally pregnant!

After you have cheered, danced and wept tears of joy, you now want to prepare for a comfortable pregnancy and the safe delivery of a healthy baby.

Because you have been following the plan and recommendations in this book, you are hopefully feeling healthier than you have for years.

I hope that you now understand how important nutrition is, alongside the marvels of IVF technology. Nutrition continues to play a vital role in your pregnancy and the healthy development of your baby. In the early weeks and months of pregnancy, the baby's cells divide and multiply rapidly and its organs are formed. Therefore, I urge you to continue your nutritional programme during pregnancy.

You may think that babies in the womb are insulated in a protective environment – that this is nature's way of protecting the next generation. But this is only true up to a point. As discussed earlier in this book, more and more research is showing that what happens to an expectant mother – what she eats or doesn't eat, for instance – has a profound effect on her baby's health now and in the future.

Fortunately, following such a healthy preconception preparation plan may help reduce the risk of having a baby who is underweight, premature or born with malformations.

A thorough discussion on maintaining optimal health of both the mother and the developing baby during pregnancy would be as long as this book. However, to get you started, refer to the following guidelines for what to include and what to avoid in your diet during pregnancy.

What to include

- ✓ An abundance of vegetables and moderate amounts of fruit
- ✓ 4-5 serves of various sources of clean organic protein foods (chicken, lean beef, eggs, wild-caught fish, legumes and beans, yoghurt, seeds (including quinoa) and nuts – except peanuts)
- ✓ Wholegrains (rice, buckwheat, millet, oats and wholegrain breads)

- ✓ Good fats (monounsaturated olive oil, coconut oil, avocado)
- ✓ 2-3 litres of filtered water a day
- ✓ Salt (Celtic, Himalayan) 1/8-1/4 teaspoon per day.

Eat every three hours to help maintain healthy blood sugar levels and ease any morning sickness.

What to avoid

- × Any foods that may harbour the bacteria Listeria monocytogenes. It usually has no effect on healthy people, but in pregnant women it can lead to miscarriage or stillbirth. High-risk foods that often contain Listeria are cold foods such as paté, deli meats, pre-mixed salads (including pre-washed salad packets), soft-serve ice-cream, soft cheeses – especially unpasteurised (blue, feta, ricotta, brie, camembert), smoked seafood, and any leftovers kept in the refrigerator for more than 12 hours. Listeria can be killed by cooking, so you can eat some pasteurised soft cheeses or smoked salmon if cooked in a quiche or pie.
- × Raw meat, raw chicken, undercooked poultry and meats, raw eggs, and raw seafood, including sushi and sashimi, as these may harbour salmonella. This can trigger miscarriage or premature birth. Foods made with raw eggs include hollandaise sauce, mayonnaise, Caesar salad dressing and semifreddo ice cream.
- × Fish with possibly high levels of mercury – such as shark, swordfish, king mackerel and tuna – and industrial pollutants from contaminated water sources.
- × Shellfish – there is a risk of contamination with Listeria, toxoplasmosis and salmonella.
- × Allergenic foods – avoid/limit any foods which cause an allergy or sensitivity in you, the baby's father or your other children.
- × Artificial sweeteners - it is best to avoid artificial food additives as much as possible during pregnancy.

- × Sugar and refined carbohydrates e.g. refined foods, white flour products and cakes. These can cause excessive weight gain, may reduce intake of nutritious foods and can increase the risk of gestational diabetes.
- × Acidic, fatty and spicy foods. These can aggravate morning sickness and heartburn.
- × Caffeine e.g. coffee, tea, cocoa, cola-type drinks and chocolate. Caffeine is a stimulant and has been linked to miscarriage. Tannins in tea can inhibit the absorption of some minerals including iron.

Also avoid:

- × Alcohol – there is NO safe limit of recreational alcohol consumption in pregnancy. Frequent and heavy drinking is associated with impaired foetal development and can result in foetal alcohol syndrome.
- × Smoking – can cause impaired growth and development.
- × Recreational drugs – causes severe damage to embryo.
- × Certain over-the-counter or prescribed pharmaceutical medications – check with your doctor and pharmacist.
- × Toxic chemicals – avoid exposure to chemicals including cleaning products and toxic products. Use safe and natural cleaning, home and personal care products.

Other lifestyle tips in early pregnancy

- Get plenty of rest.
- Take care with aerobic exercise for the first 12 weeks – your body needs time to adapt to being pregnant.
- Be careful not to increase your core body temperature as this can damage the developing foetus. Avoid electric blankets and saunas, for example.
- Don't have sex until after 12 weeks, especially if you have a high risk of miscarrying.
- Be cautious about flying in the first 12 weeks, especially long haul and if you have a high risk of miscarrying.

Supplements for pregnancy

As long as all is well, a general supplement programme for pregnancy support may include:

- A good prenatal supplement preferably containing bioactive folate, iodine, iron and vitamin D.
- Additional doses of individual nutritional supplements may be prescribed by your naturopath or doctor if deficient. For example, magnesium may be required if you suffer from leg cramps, and calcium for backache.
- Vitamin D* - additional 800-2000IU per day may be recommended (dose dependant on blood test results).
- Omega-3 DHA fish oil supplement (DHA is necessary for foetal development, especially their developing nervous system, brain, eyes and spine). In the prevention of miscarriage, Omega-3 at 4000mg per day improves uterine blood flow. Recommended dose: 1000-5000mg per day providing DHA 600-800mg and EPA 1000-1200mg.
- Probiotics, especially Lactobacillus Rhamnosus, if there is a history of allergies and eczema in either partner. Best taken daily during the last two months of pregnancy and during breastfeeding.

*A study found, at the end of pregnancy, 90 per cent of all women who were taking prenatal vitamins were still clinically deficient in vitamin D.

An analysis of vitamin D levels among daily users of prenatal supplements suggested that twice the Dietary Reference Intake of vitamin D for pregnancy and lactation was not enough to raise vitamin D levels sufficiently.

It is advisable to assess and correct vitamin D levels before conception and reassess at 12-weekly intervals during pregnancy, despite the amount of sunlight exposure and vitamin D intake.

Holick MF. High prevalence of vitamin D inadequacy and implications for health. Mayo Clin Proc. 2006; 81: 353–73.

Your doctor or naturopath may prescribe additional supplements and perhaps herbs (which are safe during pregnancy) if applicable.

Herbs have to be used with caution once you are pregnant. There are some that are especially useful in the late stages of pregnancy (raspberry leaf, for example). But once you are pregnant, it is important to only take herbs with professional advice.

Conclusion

I hope this book has encouraged you not to give up hope, to recognise that there are natural, holistic therapies to maximise your chances of IVF success, and to help make your dream of becoming pregnant one day come true, and to hopefully go on to deliver a beautiful, healthy baby.

As your doctor will also say, sadly there is no guarantee that either IVF or any of the holistic therapies mentioned in this book will work and will place a baby in your arms.

But I dearly hope and pray you will be blessed one day with the baby you so desire.

IVF is a profound procedure that is a blessing to have available. Move forward feeling encouraged, empowered and nourished on your journey.

Live well, take courage and support from others who know what path you are taking, and I hope each day brings you the strength you need to move forward in the direction of your dream to have a healthy, beautiful baby.

Jenny Blondel

MRN. ND. Dip Nut. Dip BM. Dip Hom. Dip RM.

Naturopath and fertility expert

Notes

The Diet Guide

FOR MEN

Naturopath & Fertility Expert
JENNY BLONDEL
MRN. ND. Dip Nut. Dip BM. Dip Hom. Dip RM.

Contents

Introduction

It takes 'two to tango' as they say, so it stands to reason that men's health and 'plumbing' need to be considered in the quest for a couple to become pregnant and to have a healthy baby. This is whether conception is achieved naturally or by Assisted Reproductive Technologies (ART), including IVF and Intra Cytoplasmic Sperm Injection (ICSI).

In many situations, the causes of infertility are due to a complex interaction of issues such as low sperm count in men and poor egg production in women. The way in which the sperm and the egg interact also indicates the sperm must be healthy enough to contribute to the development of an embryo.

This bonus guide is designed to help men improve their sperm health and maximise the chances of conception and support the development of a healthy embryo.

Men can support their partner, improve their sperm health and increase the chances of conception by following an **IVF Preconception Preparation Plan.** There is much research to indicate that changing lifestyle and dietary habits and taking vitamin supplements can have a positive impact on sperm production and outcomes in IVF and ICSI.

The improvement in sperm quality as a result of dietary changes and naturopathic medicine can be quite dramatic and can be seen within just a few months. Patients who have followed my IVF Preconception Preparation Plan for Men have seen a massive 500 per cent increase in sperm count in just three months.

In addition to dietary recommendations, there are specific nutritional supplements, herbal medicine and other holistic therapies to assist sperm production and support the development of quality sperm.

Apart from the benefit of helping achieve a pregnancy, your general health will almost certainly improve. In fact, many men report that by following the IVF Preconception Preparation Plan, they have more energy, fewer headaches, better digestion and feel more relaxed. Other health problems may also be resolved.

Thanks to medical research and technology advancements, there are many ways to diagnose, assist and treat male fertility problems. The diet, lifestyle and naturopathic advice in this book complement conventional medical treatments.

Support your partner and join her in a preconception preparation plan to provide 'sustenance' for your swimmers and enjoy better health along the way!

This book is dedicated to helping you regain your health and boost your fertility so you and your partner may one day hold a beautiful healthy baby in your arms.

Yours in health,

Jenny Blondel

MRN. ND. Dip Nut. Dip BM. Dip Hom. Dip RM.

Naturopath and fertility expert

CAUSES OF MALE INFERTILITY

Male factors contribute to as much as 68 to 75 per cent of infertility, and 40 per cent of those seeking Assisted Reproductive Technologies (ART), including IVF and Intra Cytoplasmic Sperm Injection (ICSI).

Approximately 40 to 50 per cent of male infertility causes are unknown, likely due to issues with sperm health (sperm quality, motility, count and sometimes the absence of sperm) and possibly ageing.

Primary (known) causes of male infertility account 30 to 40 per cent of cases. These include hormone imbalance, congenital or developmental testicular disorders (e.g. Klinefelter syndrome), undescended testes and certain medications.

Other causes may include:

- Mumps
- Testicular trauma
- Chromosome defects
- Elevated homocysteine levels
- Poor nutritional status
- Use of recreational drugs
- Pesticide exposure
- Infections including herpes and sexually transmitted infections
- Radiation
- Varicocele
- Tumour
- Excessive heat
- Heavy metal toxicity
- Cigarette smoking
- High intake of cottonseed oil
- Environmental oestrogen (xenoestrogen) exposure

Glossary of Terms

Sperm quality: The measurable parameters of semen including sperm count, motility, morphology and volume.

Sperm motility: The percentage of sperm moving.

Sperm count: The number of sperm in an ejaculate. Also referred to as sperm concentration and given as the number of sperm per millilitre.

Sperm morphology: A semen analysis factor that indicates the number or percentage of sperm in a sample that appears to have been formed normally.

Sperm progression: The quality of the movement of sperm (graded 1-4, with 1 being the highest grade).

Some sperm issues affecting fertility

Sperm are actually more vulnerable than eggs, being smaller and fully exposed physically, whereas eggs are cocooned safely within the woman's body and mature (rather than fully generate) only in the preconception months. Problems with sperm may be due to a host of reasons.

Sperm motility

Sperm must be able to move forward (or 'swim') through cervical mucous to reach an egg. A high percentage of sperm that cannot swim properly may impair a man's ability to father a child. Factors that impact motility include sperm antibody production, structural problems with the sperm tail, autoimmune disease, infection, lack of (mitochondrial) energy to propel the sperm, medication, alcohol and other toxins that affect semen quality.

Sperm vitality

This may decline due to genital tract infections or sperm antibodies. Testing for sperm antibodies is usually conducted if greater than 75 per cent of sperm are dead.

Sperm morphology

Sperm shape is an important predictive indicator of sperm-fertilising ability. Morphology is performed using the Tygerberg method of assessment. It is based on a percentage. Two per cent is needed to perform IVF. In a nutshell, shape determines success!

Agglutination

This is when sperm clump together in a circle, going nowhere. This can be caused by an infection or by antibodies.

Infection/immune issues

Infections of the prostate and epididymis (tubular structure on top of each of the testes, into which secretions drain) can interfere with sperm production or block the exit of sperm from the body. Other infections such as mumps orchitis (an inflammation of the testicles following the mumps) can result in permanent infertility.

The presence of white blood cells or bacteria indicates a genital tract infection that must be treated. It is also essential to assess the female partner to prevent cross-infection.

Herpes infection may contribute to infertility

In a study, the ejaculate from men whose wives had a history of miscarriage or implantation failure was examined for Herpes Simplex Virus (HSV). HSV was detected in the sperm of 65 per cent of the sample. The study concluded that sperm infected with HSV can have a negative effect on the course of pregnancy and/or embryo viability.

Bocharova EN, Bragina EE et al. Urologila 2007; May-June (3): 59-63

Sperm antibodies

These attach to the surface of the sperm and reduce their life span and impair semen motility and the ability to penetrate the partner's cervical mucous. It's a bit like being stuck in jelly. Antibodies on the head sperm may prevent the sperm fertilising the egg. It is important to always check for sperm antibodies. ICSI is usually performed if the percentage of sperm antibodies is greater than 90 per cent. Your IVF doctor will try, but this problem is not always easily fixed.

DNA fragmentation

It is normal for up to one in five (20 per cent) sperm to have some DNA fragmentation. Up to 85 per cent of sperm are protected from damage as the chromosomes are bound by protamines into a condensed structure. If more than 20 per cent of sperm have DNA damage, there is an increased risk of infertility, poor egg fertilisation, impaired embryo development, high implantation failure, miscarriage and recurrent miscarriage (up to three to four times higher), and genetic disease or childhood cancer in the next generation.

Ageing

Older men produce more sperm with DNA damage. This may be due to various factors including increased oxidative stress. It is even more important for older dads-to-be to follow a preconception preparation plan, including detoxification, healthy dietary changes and the use of antioxidant supplements.

Diabetes

Glandular diseases such as diabetes can interfere with hormonal control (lowers testosterone levels); sperm production; erectile function (by affecting the health of small blood vessels); ejaculate volume; and sex drive. The good news is there are successful medical treatments to address these complications.

Thyroid gland problems

Men can be subject to an underactive thyroid (hypothyroidism) just like women, which can impact on male reproductive health and fertility.

Thyroid hormone activity can affect sperm production as a large number of thyroid hormone receptors are present in the sertoli cells of the testes. These cells are responsible for nurturing healthy sperm.

Low thyroid function can result in reduced testosterone production, low sex drive, erectile dysfunction, poor testicular function and reduced sperm numbers and activity.

Gluten sensitivity

Gluten sensitivity may be linked to low sperm count, motility and morphology.

High homocysteine levels

High homocysteine levels may contribute to lowered sperm count.

Excessive heat

An increased scrotal temperature of only 1°C has been shown to decrease sperm count by about 15 per cent.

Pharmaceutical drugs

Certain medications can affect sperm quality, quantity and motility, as well as sex drive. Examples include: non-steroidal anti-inflammatory drugs (NSAIDS), tetracyclines, erythromycin and sulphur antibiotics, sulfasalazine, anabolic steroids, narcotics, cyclosporine, lithium, and H1 receptor antagonists, to name a few. Speak to your doctor if you are taking any of these medications or other medications known to impact sperm health.

Oxidative damage and exposure to toxins

Exposure to toxins can cause high levels of free radicals circulating in the body. These are chemicals that are produced naturally in the body as a by-product of a cell's metabolism. Under normal circumstances, free radicals are mopped up by the body's antioxidants. However, if they are allowed to reach high levels – sometimes due to poor diet and exposure to toxins – they can damage the DNA structure of sperm.

Other Causes of Male Infertility

Varicocele – 'varicose veins of the testes'

These are enlarged veins around the testes. They need not cause any discomfort; however, it is thought that they can overheat the testes and damage sperm production, though there are men who have varicocele and do not have any fertility problems. Unfortunately, doctors cannot predict which men with varicocele will benefit from having them treated.

Varicocele is found in up to 40 per cent of men presenting for infertility investigations. Significantly higher levels of free radicals and reduced levels of antioxidants are seen in the semen of these men.

Obstruction

Blockages in certain parts of the male reproductive system can affect fertility by stopping the sperm from being ejaculated. These blockages can occur because of scarring caused by an infection such as mycoplasma or ureaplasma, a previous surgery, or an injury (e.g. a kick to the groin while playing sport). A severe sports injury could also stop the testes producing sperm.

Undescended testes

If the testes did not come down properly after birth, then they may not be producing sperm. The incidence of this problem is increasing, and many scientists now think it is related to environmental factors. Surgery is often used to bring down a young boy's testes (which have got stuck inside the body) into the scrotum. If undescended testes are not diagnosed early enough and surgery is delayed, then a man's fertility may be compromised.

These are just some causes of male infertility. For more information, speak to your doctor or IVF/fertility clinic.

Notes

INVESTIGATIONS AND ASSESSMENTS

Since up to 50 per cent of male infertility cases may be due to inadequate sperm quality and motility, it stands to reason that men too should be investigated and assessed, preferably from the beginning when a couple are experiencing problems getting pregnant.

Your doctor will usually conduct an array of tests before referring to a specialist such as an andrologist or IVF specialist. An andrologist is a doctor that specialises in the area of male reproductive health.

Some of the tests that may be carried out include:

- Semen analysis
- Hormone test (FSH, progesterone, prolactin, LH, and androgens such as testosterone and SHBG)
- Inhibin B.

A general health screen will include:

- FBC, blood type
- LFT
- Fasting homocysteine
- Vitamin D
- Fasting lipid and glucose if appropriate
- Iron studies
- Thyroid panel
- Serum zinc and copper, selenium
- Urine analysis and sexually transmitted infection screen
- Case history to check for any trauma or previous testicular biopsy
- Erectile dysfunction, prostate problem, impotence and surgery.

They may also request:

- Genetic screening
- Testicular ultrasound
- Coeliac screen.

Your naturopath may also request:

- Nutrient and toxic element screening (e.g. aluminium, arsenic, cadmium, lead and mercury)
- Environmental impact (PCBs, pesticides, volatile solvents, phthalates, parabens, EMF radiation)
- Gluten allergy and intolerance testing
- Salivary hormone levels: DHEA, cortisol, melatonin, testosterone.

The latter tests can provide detailed information for your naturopath, taking the guesswork out of other possible contributing factors.

IVF FOR MEN

If several implantations fail, your doctor may request a Sperm Chromatin Structure Assay. This test takes a closer look at the sperm's DNA, helping to determine whether there is any fragmentation that may affect the sperm's ability to fertilise an egg or impede the development of an embryo.

If your sperm count is so low that IVF is not possible; if ejaculation does not occur; or if there is an obstruction stopping the sperm being released, your IVF clinic may use the Intra Cytoplasmic Sperm Injection (ICSI) technique, where the sperm is injected directly into the egg.

Unfortunately, this technique does not address why the sperm may have had difficulty fertilising the egg in the first place. While ICSI may make the sperm more likely to fertilise the egg and push up pregnancy rates in the process, the jury is still out as to whether the actual live birth rate has improved as a result of its popularity. ICSI, though a viable option for some couples, takes away the last bit of natural selection available through IVF.

What Happens?

Considering a female egg is invisible to the naked eye and sperm are minute in comparison to an egg, ICSI is a very delicate procedure.

For men who can't ejaculate or whose sperm are obstructed, the sperm samples are drawn off directly from the testes or epididymis. If this does not work, a biopsy is performed, in which fingernail-size pieces are taken from the testes through a tiny incision. The sperm retrieved in this way are not fully developed and may not move.

Success Rate

The average success rate for ICSI is 20 to 25 per cent, slightly higher than for IVF. This is probably due to the fact that the sperm is injected directly into the egg so the technique is not dependant on how well fertilisation takes place.

Risks

In a non-ICSI IVF cycle, approximately 100,000 sperm are placed with the egg in a Petri dish to potentially fertilise the egg to create an embryo. With ICSI however, one sperm, chosen by an IVF medical doctor or scientist, is injected into the egg. The risk of malformation is slightly increased in ICSI babies than in babies conceived naturally.

Genetic Testing

Your doctor may suggest having Karyotyping (a chromosome evaluation) before embarking on ICSI so that any genetic causes of infertility can be ruled out. If there is a genetic cause for the man's fertility, the couple are usually counselled as to whether ICSI is recommended or not because of the possibility of passing on problems to the baby.

The good news is that improvements are being made all the time, thanks to modern technology. Other techniques have been introduced to assess overall sperm health. There is now a microscope that amplifies the sperm 6,000 times. This allows a closer look at any damage to the nucleus of the sperm and therefore eliminates sperm which are more likely to cause problems.

Many healthy babies are born thanks to ART procedures such as ICSI. We are very fortunate to live in a time of such remarkable modern medicine advancements to assist fertility problems.

IVF PRECONCEPTION PREPARATION PLAN FOR MEN

There are many diet and lifestyle factors that can negatively impact the quality of the sperm, which in turn can affect you and your partner's chances of IVF success.

Smoking, too much alcohol, exposure to toxic chemicals in the workplace, recreational drug use, caffeine and a poor diet are some things that can affect sperm quality.

Sperm are manufactured in seminiferous tubules (thread-like structures which fill the two testes). Since it takes roughly 80 days for sperm to mature, a preconception preparation plan is just as important for men to prepare for an IVF cycle as it is for women.

If time permits, a preconception preparation plan for men should ideally be put in place at least three months (preferably four) before commencing IVF.

Similarly, to your partner, this comprises firstly a detox (if appropriate); followed by a new diet plan, changing lifestyle habits, taking nutritional supplements, antioxidants and herbal medicine (if applicable); and managing stress.

PRECONCEPTION DETOX FOR MEN

Male infertility is hugely influenced by environmental toxicity and radiation exposure.

Scientific and medical attention in the past decade has focused on environmental factors that may contribute to male infertility. There are several sources of radiation, chemical and environmental toxin exposure that have been directly linked to impacts on sperm health. Even more compelling is the evidence that frequent exposure to electromagnetic radiation (EMR) causes damage to sperm.

The goal is to identify those factors that may be contributing to infertility and to minimise/avoid these influences as much as possible. Some examples are listed below.

Radiation Exposure

X-rays

Exposure to ionising radiation from X-rays can affect sperm health. Jude Ford's research shows that sperm morphology can be affected by a single lower body x-ray for up to three years after the event.[45]

Microwave radiation

Microwave ovens emit an extremely large electromagnetic field and can destroy proteins and the enzymes required to absorb vitamins and minerals. Stand in the next room if you have to use a microwave.

Electromagnetic Fields (EMF) and Electromagnetic Radiation (EMR)

This is the type of radiation that enables electricity to function - it is what surrounds us when we turn on televisions, mobile phones, tablets and laptops. There are now concerns being raised about the impact of wireless network connections (WiFi) on all aspects of health, including the reproductive health of men and women.

[45] Jude Ford is an international leader in reproductive genetics and environmental toxic effects on sperm and egg health.

Increasingly, research is showing that computer use, especially in conjunction with WiFi, may be associated with a decrease in sperm motility (percentage of sperm moving) and an increase in sperm DNA damage.[46] Consider investing in a laptop 'shield', or use plants and crystals to help absorb some of the radiation.

Mobile (cell) phones

When carried close to the lower body (e.g. in trouser pockets), mobile phones can affect testicular health, including sperm count and motility. Studies have confirmed a direct link with the proximity of switched on mobile phones to the testes and the impact on sperm quality and count.[47] Leading experts from top universities further report that there is a direct relationship between duration of mobile phone use and sperm count decline. Sperm count is reduced by half in men who carry mobile phones in their trouser pockets for four hours per day.[48]

The testicular barrier that protects sperm is one of the most sensitive of tissues in the body and highly absorbent. Mitochondrial DNA of sperm is damaged three times more if exposed to mobile phone radiation.[49]

Where possible, don't carry your mobile phone in your trouser pocket. Turn them off when not in use. It's best to store mobile phones at least three feet away from your body. Don't sleep with your mobile phone in the bedroom. When left on at night, they can prevent delta wave deep sleep.

[46] Doré JF, Chignol MC et al Laptop computers with Wi-Fi decrease human sperm motility and increase sperm DNA fragmentation. Fertil Steril. 2012 Apr;97(4):e12;. Epub 2012 Feb 10.
[47] Agarwal,A et al. Fertility and Sterility 2009;92(4):1318-1325.
[48] PLoS ONE 4(7): e6446.
[49] ElectromagneticHealth.org August 29, 2013

In the bedroom

Studies link electric blankets and water beds to male fertility problems. Clock radios also give off a very large electrical field, so keep the clock radio at least one metre away from where you sleep. Try to sleep away from all other active appliances, including televisions and tablet computers. Lastly, make sure the head of your bed is not close to a fuse box, which produce electro-magnetic radiation.

Environmental Chemicals

Xenoestrogens

Xenoestrogens are synthetic oestrogens which affect the fertility of both humans and wildlife. They come from pesticides and plastics and are stored in body fat. The massive increase of xenoestrogens in our environment has coincided with a decrease in sperm counts of up to 50 per cent over the past 15 years; an increase in testicular cancer; and a doubling in the number of boys born with undescended testes.

Phthalates

Phthalates are chemicals used as solvents, lubricants, stabilisers and plasticisers. These too, have been linked to male fertility problems.

Bisphenol A

Bisphenol A (BPA) is found in the interior coating of tin cans, polystyrene cups, some dental material, and aluminium water bottles. Quantifiable levels have been found in some male IVF patients, indicating a possible link with infertility problems.[50] Try to limit exposure to BPA by avoiding canned foods, bottled water stored in BPA plastic (although many manufacturers have removed BPA from water bottles) and hot foods kept in takeaway containers,

[50] Highlights from the 64th Annual Meeting of the American Society of Reproductive Medicine. www.asm/org/media/press/AM08_bisphenol.html

Styrofoam, polystyrene and cling (plastic) wraps. Look out for plastics with recycling symbols #3 and #7.

Organochloride compounds (OCCs)

Examples of organochloride compounds (OCCs) include DDT and DDE. Exposure has been associated with reduced semen quality, contributing to male infertility and miscarriages. Exposure during fertilisation also affects the development of the embryo.[51]

Glycol ether

Glycol ether is used in surface coatings, printing inks, cleaners, chemicals used in farming, and as flow improvers in water-based paints. Exposure has been related to low motile sperm count in men attending IVF fertility clinics.[52]

Organic solvents

Organic solvents are found in textiles, paints and plastics. Laboratory workers especially are exposed to organic solvents. These too have been linked to male infertility and increased risk of malformations in a developing baby.

Heavy metals

Heavy metals such as lead, mercury, cadmium, cobalt, chromium and boron can cause adverse reproductive outcomes such as decreased sperm quality and quantity, sperm antibodies, testicular damage and central nervous system problems. Some primary sources of heavy metals are: petrochemical and gas fumes; old paint; smoking (active and passive); tools; cadmium in some paints; dental amalgams; tellurium (a by-product of welding); consumption of mercury–contaminated fish; non-stick aluminium cookware; certain antiperspirants (especially sprays that are inhaled); some antacids; and some tap water. It is important to remove these heavy metals before preconception health care begins.

[51] Tiemann U. Reprod Toxic 2008; 25:316-326.
[52] Cherry N, Moore H et al. *Occup Environ Med* 2008 April 16.

Domestic Chemicals

Domestic chemicals such as bleach, mould treatments, oven cleaners, and ammonia-based spray and wipe products are known reproductive toxins.

Instead, use alternatives such as Norwex™ (an anti-bacterial cloth system) and natural cleaning products including lemon juice, tea tree oil and baking soda.

Other domestic chemicals to avoid include products used in home renovations such as sanding lead paint, glues and varnishes; personal care products containing sodium lauryl sulfate; garden pesticides; insect sprays; and chlorine.

Conduct a domestic chemical evaluation and discard toxic products from your kitchen, bathroom, garage, tool/workshop and garden.

Recreational Chemicals

There are plenty of chemicals in your recreational environment such as chlorinated swimming pools. Chlorine is a known hormone disruptor, especially in regard to thyroid health, indirectly affecting male fertility.

Golf courses are also saturated with pesticides and fertilisers, which is why golfers have a higher incidence of breast and prostate cancer. The levels of these chemicals are also higher in the warm early morning hours when the humidity is at its peak, a popular time for golfers.

Naturopathic Detox

Enhancing liver detoxification pathways and optimising antioxidant status is important to reduce the toxic burden of many chemicals, as is eating a healthy, wholefood, antioxidant-rich diet.

Your naturopath may recommend:

- Amino acids such as glutamine, glycine, taurine, cysteine, methionine and choline. These are often found combined in many specific detox formulas
- Chelators such as humic acid, vitamin C and glutathione
- Herbs such as Coriander, Garlic, Milk Thistle, Rosemary, Schizandra and Turmeric to support liver detoxification
- Superfoods such as chlorella, spirulina, blue-green algae, wheatgrass, bee pollen, royal jelly, hemp and goji berries
- A detox drink such as my detox cocktail
- Oil pulling
- Avoiding chemical exposure, including smoking cigarettes and cannabis
- Lifestyle changes to minimise chemical and radiation exposure.

More information on Preconception Detox can be found in Section 2 of *Making Babies: The Holistic IVF Diet Guide.*

PRECONCEPTION AND IVF DIET PLAN FOR MEN

A balanced diet consisting of health-promoting foods is not only essential for overall health, but also for optimal sperm health.

A diet rich in red meat and refined grains (think white flour, white bread, wraps and baked goods) can significantly reduce sperm motility, which is critical for sperm to effectively penetrate and fertilise the egg.

Study: Sperm motility may improve with a healthy diet

A healthy diet can lead to more motile sperm. This is the outcome of a study presented at the American Society of Reproductive Medicine, which analysed two styles of diet; one being 'Western' (lots of red meat and refined carbohydrates including white flour products such as sweets and soft drinks), or 'Prudent' (Mediterranean-type diet high in fish, fruit, vegetables, legumes, wholegrains, healthy fats and oils). The men following the Mediterranean-style diet had significantly greater sperm motility.

The findings support that a diet rich in fruits, vegetables, chicken, fish, wholegrains and healthy fats may be an inexpensive and safe way to improve at least one measure of semen quality.

If you and your partner are about to commence IVF, it's time to cut out the French fries, soft drinks and fast food, and increase your intake of fruits and vegetables, grass-fed meats, oily fish, nuts, seeds, beans, eggs, and healthy fats such as avocado.

Fertility and Sterility, Gaskins A, et al "Dietary patterns and semen quality in young men" Fertility Sterility 2011; 90(3) Suppl: Abstract O-27. Human Reproduction, Volume 27, Issue 11, (October 2012), p. 2899-2907.

Consuming a Mediterranean-style diet that focuses on whole, unprocessed foods such as wholegrains, vegetables, fruits, quality protein, healthy fats, nuts and seeds provides a reasonable supply of antioxidant nutrients essential for sperm health (see box).

What to Eat Everyday

Vegetables

Eat vegetables such as asparagus, aubergines, bok choy, broccoli, brussels sprouts, cabbage, carrots, courgettes, leafy greens, peppers, pumpkin, spinach, sweet potato, garlic, onion and culinary herbs. **Salad vegetables** such as avocado, cucumber, lettuce, mung beans, rocket, watercress and tomatoes are also great.

Fruits

Include fruits such as berries, apples, bananas, pears, melons, plums, apricots, red grapes, mangoes and pink grapefruit in your meal plan. Preferably choose organic fruit and vegetables and eat what is in season.

Legumes

Eat legumes such as beans, pulses, chickpeas and lentils.

Quality protein

Insufficient protein in the diet will cause poor sperm quality, morphology and motility. The entire sperm (head, body and tail) is dependent on protein, so include grass-fed meats, fish, organic chicken, organic dairy foods (if tolerant) and free range, organic eggs in your diet.

Nuts and seeds

Snack on almonds, Brazil nuts, hazelnuts, macadamia nuts, pecans, walnuts, pumpkin seeds and sunflower seeds. Just 4g of walnuts a day for 12 weeks has been shown to increase sperm parameters by 75 per cent!

Healthy fats

Rich in essential fatty acids, healthy fats include avocado, coconut oil, flaxseeds, and oily fish like salmon, sardines and mackerel.

Zinc-rich foods

Zinc is important for sperm health and controlling and maintaining healthy testosterone levels. Zinc can be found in oysters (which contain the highest amounts of zinc of any food), pumpkin seeds, animal protein, wholegrains and leafy green vegetables (although the latter depends on the mineral density of the soil quality where the vegetables are grown).

Green tea

Research shows that consumption of green tea increases the levels of antioxidants in the blood. The antioxidants in the tea help protect DNA in the maturing sperm.

Filtered water

Since sperm are manufactured and spend time in a fluid environment i.e. semen, hydration is paramount. Drink at least two litres of filtered or spring water daily.

Superfoods

Green superfood drinks are an excellent choice to add to a preconception diet. You can either make your own drink by blending barley grass, wheatgrass, spirulina, carrots and apples. Such superfood drinks contain antioxidants, complex carbohydrates, vitamins, minerals, trace minerals, and vegetarian protein.

A green superfood drink like this is a great choice for men whose diets are low in fresh fruits and green vegetables. The nutrients are rapidly delivered to all the body systems for an energy boost that can often be felt immediately. It offers a natural pick-me-up without caffeine or artificial stimulants.

More information on superfoods can be found in Section 4, of *Making Babies: The Holistic IVF Diet Guide.*

What to Avoid

The following is a list of foods that are known to affect male reproductive health and damage sperm.

Bad fats

Bad fats come from sources such as saturated fats, hydrogenated oils, trans-fatty acids, cottonseed and palm oils. Avoid margarine, the fats of meat, and fried foods. These all promote free radical damage.

Cottonseed oil may contain toxic residues because of the heavy spraying of cotton and its high levels of gossypol, a substance known to inhibit sperm function.

Excess dairy

Studies suggest dairy products, particularly those with full-fat content, may have an adverse effect on semen quality as they are often high in xenoestrogens. If you are having dairy, then at least opt for organic milk and butter. Go easy on cheese, cream, ice-cream and custard.

Soy products

Excess soy intake can lead to hormonal imbalances in men as well as women. Choose non-genetically modified, organic and preferably fermented forms of soy.

Refined sugar

Sweets, candy, sweet biscuits, doughnuts and soft drinks are detrimental to not just your sperm health, but your waist line too - not to mention the knock-on effect on inflammation, blood sugar health, blood lipids (cholesterol and triglycerides) and heart health. Avoid or limit the intake of such refined foods and opt for low sugar and low glycaemic index foods.

Artificial foods

Food preservatives, colourings and additives are no good for anyone and should be avoided where possible.

Alcohol

Excessive alcohol intake is detrimental to sperm quality. Limit or ideally avoid alcohol during the three or four preconception months until your sperm sample is required for IVF or ICSI.

Caffeine

Caffeine is found in coffee, energy drinks, black tea and green tea. Excessive consumption is linked to lower sperm counts, poor sperm quality and motility. In fact, more than 300mg of caffeine per day can result in a 20 per cent higher risk of DNA damage to sperm than for men with no caffeine intake.

Gut Health and Male Fertility

A healthy gut microbiome balance is important for reproductive and hormone health in both men and women. The microbiome can affect hormone health as gut bacteria is important for metabolism and excretion of hormones, acting like a second liver (the liver is the most important organ for processing hormones). If applicable, your naturopath can provide dietary advice, digestive enzymes, prebiotics and specific probiotics to help achieve and maintain a healthy gut microbiome.

In addition, food allergies/intolerances need to be addressed and managed. Your naturopath can arrange or conduct testing to see if this is an issue and assist in the management of any allergies/intolerances.

An acidic pH in the gut can also contribute to inflammation, heartburn, acid reflux, fatigue and sore joints. Eating alkaline foods can assist in balancing pH.

Inflammatory bowel diseases and gastrointestinal diseases such as coeliac disease are linked to malabsorption issues and reduced semen quality, often because the body is not absorbing the nutrients it needs to sustain optimal gut and immune health. Once again, your naturopath can advise dietary therapy and nutritional and herbal medicine to assist in managing such conditions.

PRECONCEPTION LIFESTYLE ADVICE FOR MEN

Lifestyle factors such as smoking; the use of recreational drugs; weight gain; lack of exercise or the wrong type of exercise; overheating (e.g. sweating it out in saunas); poor sleep; and certain medications can significantly impact on male fertility, including issues with testosterone levels and sperm health.

Testosterone

The hormone known as testosterone plays a key role in the overall health of men. Testosterone is produced in the Leydig cells. This hormone is responsible for changes that occur around puberty, resulting in body and facial hair and a deep voice. Testosterone is needed for sex drive and helping achieve and maintain an erection. It also helps maintain bone density and muscle mass.

Testosterone levels generally reach their peak during early adulthood and continue to drop a little with each passing year. Low testosterone levels can impact adversely on men's fertility.

While there's no magical solution for replacing actual testosterone levels you once had at age 20, there are effective solutions that may greatly help your efforts overall. These include maintaining an ideal weight, cutting out refined carbs, getting enough sleep, eating zinc-rich foods and talking to your doctor about safe testosterone treatments such as natural bio-identical hormone replacement therapy.

Smoking

There is a strong association between smoking and reduced sperm health, including count, quality, motility and morphology. Smoking by either partner reduces the success rate of IVF. It also greatly reduces the levels of vitamin C, an important antioxidant required for sperm health.

What's more, the consequence of Dad smoking lowers his potential daughters' Anti-Mullerian Hormone (AMH) levels! An AMH reading is considered a useful hormone marker for predicting ovarian reserve and ageing.

Quitting smoking will not only benefit your reproductive health but general health as well.

Marijuana

Smoking marijuana can reduce testosterone levels and negatively impact sperm quality. Stopping smoking marijuana will not only benefit your reproductive health but general health as well.

In addition, other recreational drugs e.g. ecstasy, cocaine, heroin and anabolic steroids should be completely avoided. Speak to your doctor if this is an issue for you.

Maintain a Healthy Weight

Overweight men with pre-diabetes tendencies most likely have significantly lower testosterone levels. The more fat a man has, the more oestrogen produced, decreasing testosterone production. Studies show that low testosterone levels and diabetes are strongly linked.

Excess refined sugar can decrease testosterone levels as much as 30 per cent. This is true whether you have diabetes, pre-diabetes, or are normal in terms of glucose tolerance. Cutting out all forms of sugar such as sweets, chocolate, biscuits and doughnuts will also go a long way to trimming down the waistline.

What's more, obesity has a detrimental effect on sperm motility and erectile function. The best way to reach and maintain a normal healthy weight is to regularly exercise and eat a nutritious calorie-controlled diet. Cutting out alcohol and refined carbohydrates, consuming adequate protein throughout the day and observing portion sizes may be all it takes from a dietary perspective to lose the spare tyre.

Refer to Section 3 of *Making Babies: The Holistic IVF Diet Guide* for detailed information on weight management.

Exercise

Exposure to heat (e.g. wetsuits, saunas, spas, tight Lycra cycling pants) and pressure such as bike riding has been shown to decrease sperm health and been associated with prostatitis (swelling and inflammation of the prostate gland). In fact, cycling more than five hours per week has been associated with low sperm concentrations.[53]

Exercising in a way that creates too much heat and physical pressure on the testes is not helpful. It is better to go for a brisk 20-minute walk and do some weight-bearing exercise for 20 minutes daily.

In one study, researchers found that men who exercised more than 15 hours per week had 73 per cent higher sperm concentrations compared to men who exercised less than five hours per week. The study also found that men who spent more than 20 hours per week watching television had 44 per cent lower sperm counts compared to men who did not watch any television.[54]

So, get moving, with the exception of too much cycling! And lastly, don't finish an exercise session by resting in a warm spa or sweating it out in a hot sauna. This will raise your body and scrotal temperature, impacting sperm health further...

[53] Wise La, Cramer DW, Hornstein MD, et al. Physical activity and semen quality among men attending an infertility clinic. Fertil Steril 2011; 95:1025-30.
[54] Gaskins AJ, Mediola J, Afeiche M, et al. Br J Sports Med Published Online First: 4 February 2013 doi:10.1136/bjsports-2012-091644.

Keep Cool

The male reproductive organs are outside the body for a good reason. The testes need to be a few degrees cooler than body temperature (37°C/98.4°C) because sperm production is most efficient at 34°C (93.2°F). Anything that brings the testes closer to the body, raising their temperature, may affect sperm count. Average scrotal temperatures in humans are typically 2.5 to 3 degrees Celsius lower than body temperature.

Keep testes cool by avoiding hot baths, saunas, heated car seats and wearing tight-fitting underwear (including cycling pants), all of which can increase scrotal temperature. Also avoid using electric blankets in bed.

Sleep

Adequate sleep helps all aspects of health, including physical, mental and emotional wellbeing. Researchers agree that a lack of sleep can significantly reduce testosterone levels even in healthy young men. In fact, the effects are obvious after just one week of decreased sleep.

The majority of men need anywhere from seven to nine hours each night for optimal health so aim for eight hours per night, getting to bed ideally no later than 10.30pm.

Medications

Always discuss with your doctor any medications you are taking, have taken or plan to take, as they can affect sperm health and semen production.

For more information on lifestyle recommendations, refer to Section 6 of *Making Babies: The Holistic IVF Diet Guide.*

Notes

NUTRITIONAL MEDICINE FOR IVF AND MALE FERTILITY

Apart from diet and lifestyle changes, nutritional medicine can significantly improve sperm health. Several studies have shown the beneficial effects of specific vitamins, minerals, amino acids and antioxidant treatment on sperm parameters. Such supplementation may help with IVF outcomes, even to the point where less invasive treatments could become an option.

Sperm is produced 24 hours a day, seven days a week. Since sperm formation takes approximately 80 days, it will usually take at least this amount of time before the benefits from a nutrient medicine programme are felt. Ideally you should begin the programme three months before starting IVF.

Antioxidants for Sperm Health

Men exposed to higher levels of sources of free radicals are much more likely to have abnormal sperm and sperm counts. Free radical or oxidative damage to sperm is thought to be responsible for many cases of male infertility, with 40 per cent higher levels found in infertile men.

> Human sperm are the worst in the animal kingdom (compared to baboons which have 90 per cent good sperm).

Antioxidants such as vitamins C and E, Lycopene, Grape Seed, Coenzyme Q10 and Alpha Lipoic acid are necessary to protect the DNA within the head of the sperm. They promote survival and longevity of sperm and enable it to detect the signals from recently ovulated egg.

Researchers conclude that there is sufficient evidence that antioxidant supplementation in men improves the outcome of live births and pregnancy rates for couples undergoing IVF cycles.[55]

[55] Showell MG, Brown J, Tazdani A, Stankiewicz MT, Hart RJ, Antioxidants for male subfertility, the Cochrane Library, 2011, Issue, 2, Whey Publishers.

Nutritional Requirements for Healthy Sperm

The **head** of the tadpole-like sperm carries the genetic material which will enter the egg and join the female genetic material. The head of the sperm has to contain certain enzymes and be hard enough to penetrate the egg.

The one issue that a semen analysis does not identify is whether the sperm can get into the egg and fertilise it. Sometimes the head of the sperm is not strong enough to penetrate the egg. This is where you may be advised to have ICSI treatment, which involves inserting the sperm directly into the egg. However, the key nutrients provided in a nutritional supplement may strengthen the head and neck of the sperm and help it penetrate the egg.

The middle part of the sperm provides the energy needed by the tail to move forward. It also contains the DNA that plays a part in gene inheritance. Key nutrients are required for the energy-producing cells, the mitochondria, to work.

The tail of the sperm needs to be strong to make the sperm swim in the right direction and, once again, is fuelled by key nutrients.

A single sperm comprises the following key nutritional ingredients:

- Protein
- Essential fatty acids and vitamin E
- Selenium
- Coenzyme Q10 (neck)
- Antioxidants (head, neck)
- B vitamins
- Vitamin D3
- Calcium
- Hydration: sperm like to swim in nice fluid, not jelly!

Based on this information, scientific research and clinical evidence, nutritional supplements that can assist male reproductive health include the following.

Vitamins

Vitamin A and Beta-carotene

Vitamin A and Beta-carotene are necessary for the health of the testes and sperm production. Low concentrations of vitamin A are associated with abnormal semen parameters, while beta-carotene levels are significantly lower in infertile men with immune issues. Supplemental Beta-carotene improves sperm concentration and motility. Recommended dose: up to 30,000IU, particularly if there are issues with mucous membrane health.

B vitamins

B vitamins (especially folate and B12) are required for healthy sperm and gene synthesis (DNA and RNA) and expression. Folate (vitamin B9) and B12 are concentrated within the head of the sperm but provide vital nutrients for sperm generation and survival. Recommended dose: 1-2 doses of a high strength bioactive B complex per day.

Folate

Folate is important for sperm production due to its role in cell division and DNA synthesis. Low levels of folate are linked with increased sperm DNA damage[56] and elevated homocysteine.[57] Supplementation has been shown to improve sperm count.[58] Recommended dose: 500IU per day unless your tests show you are methylenetetrahydrofolate reductase (MTHFR) homozygous positive, then 1mg 5-MTHFR (active form of folate) per day.

[56] Sinclair S. Male Infertility: nutritional and environmental considerations Althern Med 2000 Feb;5(1):28-38.

[57] "Low folate in seminal plasma is associated with increased sperm DNA damage," Boxmeer JC, Smit M, et al, Fertil Steril, 2009; 92(2): 548-56.

[58] Wong et al. The New England Journal of Medicine 2002; 344(15): 1172-1173.

Vitamin B12

Vitamin B12 is needed to maintain healthy blood, energy levels and fertility. Low levels have been associated with lower sperm count, poor motility and increased sperm abnormalities.[59] Higher doses of vitamin B12 in some studies have demonstrated significant improvement in sperm count. Recommended dose: from 100IU up to 6000IU per day may be required to improve sperm count.

Vitamin C

Vitamin C improves all semen parameters. Even a marginal deficiency causes oxidative damage to sperm, resulting in reduced sperm motility and viability. Supplementation improves sperm viability and motility and reduces abnormal sperm.[60] Sperm quality in smokers will improve in proportion with the level of vitamin C supplementation.

In one study, 30 infertile but otherwise healthy men received either 200mg or 1000mg of vitamin C or a placebo daily. Sperm count, viability, motility and other parameters were measured weekly. After one week, the 1000mg group demonstrated a 140 per cent increase in sperm count; the 200mg group a 112 per cent increase, and the placebo group no change. At the end of 60 days, all of the vitamin C groups had impregnated their wives, compared with none of the placebo group.[61]

This vitamin is 'not negotiable' – it should be part of every man's fertility supplement programme. In fact, men should take it all the time! Recommended dose: up to 1g every three hours especially if there are problems with the head of the sperm. Otherwise 2-3g divided dose per day.

[59] Boxmeer JC et al. J Androl. 2007; 28(4):521-7.
[60] Akmal M, Qadri JQ, Al Waili NS, Thangal S, Haq A, Saloom KY: Improvement in human semen quality after oral supplementation of vitamin C. J Med Food, 2006 Fall; 9(3): 440-2.
[61] Dawsen EB, Harris WA, Rankin WE, et al. Effect of ascorbic acid on male fertility. Ann NY Acad Sci 1987; 598:312-323.

Vitamin D (3)

A deficiency in vitamin D (3) is associated with lower sperm parameters. It is involved in protecting sperm DNA, enabling sperm movement, and assisting the sperm to 'find' the egg. It also provides an autoimmune mechanism to protect against sperm antibodies. It is found in the head and neck of the sperm. Vitamin D is a fat-soluble vitamin, which comes mainly from exposure to sunlight and certain foods such as cod liver oil, oily fish, egg yolks and mushrooms. Exposing the skin to the midday sun for 20 to 30 minutes produces about 2000IU of vitamin D. Recommended dose: 1000-10000IU per day depending on pathology results.

Vitamin E

Vitamin E is another crucial vitamin as it is the main antioxidant for cell membranes that surround the sperm. It protects the delicate DNA within the sperm from damage and has been shown to improve sperm motility.

Vitamin E enhances the ability of sperm to fertilise an egg in an IVF setting. What's more, beneficial results have also been observed in patients undergoing ICSI.[62]

Recommended dose: 500-1500IU mixed combination per day. Vitamin E when taken with selenium (150-250mcg per day) significantly improves sperm quality than just vitamin E on its own.

[62] Aitken Rj, Clarkson JS, Hargreave TB, et al. Analysis of the relationship between defective sperm function and the generation of reactive oxygen species in cases of oligozoospermia. J Androl 1989; 10:214-220.

Minerals

Calcium

Calcium is a key component of seminal fluid and supports and nourishes the sperm. It is involved in sperm motility and enhancing 'proper' sperm swimming, which is important for fertilisation. Recommended dose: 800mg per day.

Selenium

Selenium is an essential mineral for treating male infertility. It is a potent antioxidant and important for the overall health of the sperm, including sperm maturation and motility. It is also important for testosterone synthesis.

High concentrations are found in the tail, but also throughout the body of the sperm. The tail of the sperm should have a 'whip-like' action. If they are low in selenium, the sperm will swim around in circles rather than forwards (thereby not fertilising the egg). A deficiency of selenium can also cause deterioration in the quality and motility of semen.[63]

Studies show that 200mcg of selenium taken in combination with 600mg of n-acetyl-cysteine (NAC) per day can improve overall semen parameters. However, once supplementation stopped, parameters reverted back to their baseline readings.[64] Recommended dose: 200mcg per day; however, if there is poor motility, up to 300mcg may be prescribed per day (based on a weight of 65kg).

[63] Journal Trace Elem Med Biol. 2015 Jan; 29:31-8

[64] Safaromejad MR, Safarinejad S; Efficacy of selenium &/or N-acetyl-cysteine for improving semen parameters in infertile men: a double-blind, placebo controlled, randomised study J Urol, 2009 Feb, 18(2): 741-51. Epub 2008 Dec 16.

Zinc

Zinc is perhaps the most critical trace mineral for male sexual function. It is involved in virtually every aspect of male reproduction, including hormone metabolism (testosterone production), and sperm count, motility (important for head and neck of sperm) and morphology. It is also important for testes development and prostate health and protects sperm chromosomes from oxidative damage.[65] Because it also provides antimicrobial effects on semen, it is indicated for sperm antibody problems or underlying infections.

Zinc is found in high concentrations within semen. Approximately 2.5mg of zinc is lost per ejaculate. Zinc deficiencies lead to poor sperm count, impotence, small testes, and male infertility. Causes of deficiency may include certain drugs and medications, coeliac disease, liver or kidney disease, vegetarian and vegan diets, inflammatory bowel disease (IBD) and parasites.

Recommended dose: 30-60mg per day. However, 120mg per day may be prescribed for the first month, especially if copper levels are high. Then 90mg per day may be recommended, especially if there are early colour changes in hair (turning grey early), hair and facial hair loss. Consider a picolinate form to increase zinc status faster. If sensitive, a zinc citrate form will reduce nausea. Take zinc after meals.

[65] Reprod Biomed Online 2015 Apr;30(4):334-9

Amino Acids

L-Arginine

L-Arginine is an amino acid required for cell replication and healthy sperm formation, helping prevent sperm abnormalities. It has been shown to improve sperm count and motility. Lower levels are found when men are stressed. Recommended dose: 4000mg per day.

L-Carnitine

L-Carnitine is an amino acid derived from lysine and/or methionine. Lower amounts have been found in the sperm of infertile men. Several clinical studies have shown that carnitine supplementation can produce dramatic improvements in sperm count, motility and vitality.[66] It works synergistically with Coenzyme Q10 to improve energy production at a cellular and sperm level. It is also an effective antioxidant and benefits heart health. Recommended dose: 3000mg per day.

Essential Fatty Acids

Omega-3 fatty acids

Omega-3 fatty acids are important for sperm health as they help keep sperm fluid and flexible and may assist in the sperm's ability to fertilise an egg. Both omega-3 EPA and DHA are important. It is critical to have the right balance of fats and not too much omega-6 to omega-3 as this can impact on sperm health. Higher levels of omega-3 oils and lower consumption of saturated fats are associated with higher sperm count and quality.[67] Recommended dose: 800-1000mg of EPA per day and 400-700mg of DHA per day.

[66] Cryoprotective effect of l-carnitine on motility, vitality and DNA oxidation of human spermatozoa: Banihani S, Agarwal A, et al, Andrologia, 2013 July 3; [Epub ahead of print].
[67] "Dietary fat and semen quality among men attending a fertility clinic," Attaman JA, Toth TL, et al, Hum Reprod, 2012 Mar 13.

Antioxidants

Alpha Lipoic Acid (ALA)

Alpha Lipoic Acid (ALA) is a powerful antioxidant and provides protection both inside and outside the sperm, acting as a 'shield' for the sperm. ALA improves sperm motility and viability and helps minimise DNA damage. It may also assist with energy supply to the sperm.

ALA increases the benefits of other antioxidants such as vitamin C, vitamin E, CoenzymeQ10 and glutathione. It also helps remove heavy metals in the body. Recommended dose: 200-400mg (up to 600mg) per day. R-ALA is the preferred form.

Coenzyme Q10 (CoQ10)

Coenzyme Q10 is considered the most crucial and powerful antioxidant for sperm structure due to its role in mitochondrial energy release. It is also important for the health of all new cells, specifically sperm cells. CoQ10 is concentrated in the head and mid-pieces (neck) of the sperm. It promotes sperm motility and survival and provides optimal energy to assist the sperm's travel to the egg. Low levels are found in men with varicoceles. IVF scientists also use it in culture settings. Recommended dose: up to 600mg per day (divided dose).

Grape seed

Grape seed is an antioxidant that protects all cells in the body, including those in the testes and sperm, from oxidative (free radical) damage. It has also been shown to improve microcirculation in the testes leading to healthy sperm development.[68] Recommended dose: 6-12g equivalent of dry seed per day.

Lycopene

Lycopene is found in high concentrations in the testes and semen. Reduced levels are associated with male infertility. Human trials

[68] Dartenuc et al. Food and Chemical Toxicology 2002; 40(5):599-607.

have reported improvement in sperm parameters and pregnancy rates with supplementation of 4-8mg lycopene daily for three to 12 months.[69] Recommended dose: just 2mg twice daily over three months can improve overall sperm health. However, up to 8mg per day may be prescribed.

N-Acetylcysteine

N-Acetylcysteine (NAC) is a modified amino acid based on L-Cysteine. This compound has direct antioxidant effects and is beneficial for improving semen quality, protecting sperm and preventing DNA damage.[70] Recommended dose range: 500mg to 4000mg per day.

The good news is many of these nutrients can be obtained in a specifically formulated male reproductive multivitamin and mineral formula, with the exception of CoQ10, ALA and perhaps the amino acids. Be advised by your naturopath and/or doctor as to what you may require. Taking supplements at mealtimes may minimise stomach upset.

Nutritional medicine is always best taken under the care and guidance of your healthcare practitioner. Always consult a registered, experienced naturopath or nutritionist regarding advice on nutritional medicine.

[69] Asian J Androl. 2014 May-Jun;16(3):420-5

[70] Ciftci H, et. al. (2009). Effects of N-acetylcysteine on semen parameters and oxidative/antioxidant status. Urology. Volume 74, Issue, (pp. 173-6)

Notes

HERBAL MEDICINE FOR IVF AND MALE FERTILITY

Herbal medicine can be extremely effective in both assisting and treating male reproductive health problems. Herbs may be prescribed during the preconception months to assist healthy conception, naturally or by IVF. Some examples of herbs include the following

Astragalus

More commonly known as an immune tonic, Astragalus helps improve sperm motility. This may be valuable when treating male infertility where poor sperm motility is a suspected factor.[71]

Damiana

Damiana is indicated for low libido, erection difficulties and low mood. It also has a traditional use as a nerve tonic for depression and anxiety (particularly due to sexual issues); nervous dyspepsia (nervous upset stomach); and constipation.

Ginkgo

A highly effective circulatory stimulant, Ginkgo helps increase peripheral blood supply to the penis and overall circulation.

Gotu Kola

Gotu Kola is a remarkable healing herb - it enhances the connective tissue of the vascular wall and reduces inflammation, and is therefore indicated for conditions such as varicoceles.

Korean Ginseng

Korean Ginseng has a strong traditional use as a male tonic. It promotes the growth of the testes, raises testosterone levels and improves sperm quality. It is indicated as an energy tonic when there is lowered vitality, feeling depleted post-ejaculation and low sex drive. Note: It is not for all men, especially for those who are already 'wired'!

[71] Hong CY1, Ku J, Wu P. Et al, Astragalus membranous stimulates human sperm motility in vitro. Am J Chin Med. 1992;20(3-4):289-94.

Mucuna

Another Ayurvedic herb, Mucuna is found in powdered form (often as a superfood). It has been traditionally used for stamina and endurance, stress support, resistance against infection, mood health and male reproductive health (poor sperm health and impotence). It has shown to improve hormone levels and is prescribed to improve sperm count and motility.

Saw Palmetto

Saw Palmetto is a traditional male tonic for male reproductive health. It reduces the more potent problematic form of testosterone - di-hydrotestosterone (responsible for prostate enlargement) - which is associated with sperm defects.

Tribulus

Tribulus is the ultimate male reproductive tonic. It is known to make stronger, faster swimmers! Tribulus increases fertility, sperm virility, sperm production, and rejuvenates the reproductive system. More specifically, it increases ejaculate volume, and sperm count, concentration and motility. It has also been shown to improve conception rates where male infertility is a factor.[72] It is used to treat impotence, low sex drive and overall sexual functioning – a true herbal aphrodisiac! NB. It is important to use a Bulgarian standardised extract.

[72] Adimeoja A, Phytochemicals and the breakthrough of traditional herbs in the management of sexual dysfunctions. International Journal of Andrology Volume 23, Issue S2, Pages 82-84. Published online 4/1/2000.

Tribulus studies on male infertility and impotence

A 2006 study reported the use of Tribulus in improving sperm motility and increased penetration of cervical mucous by sperm. The five-year study involved 100 Bulgarian couples in which the men were infertile due to immune issues. Pregnancy was achieved in 44 per cent of couples.

Another study involved treating male patients with sperm motility problems after a varicocele operation with a Bulgarian Tribulus extract for 90 days. Significant improvements in sperm motility were observed as well as an increase in ejaculate quantity.

Tribulus combines well with Damiana, Korean Ginseng, Rhodiola, Saw Palmetto or Withania for male reproductive health problems, infertility and low sex drive.

Withania

Withania has a traditional use in Ayurvedic medicine as an aphrodisiac, therefore it is indicated for male sexual 'inadequacy'. It is also an adrenal adaptogen (tonic) that supports the stress response.

Your naturopath or medical herbalist may also prescribe other herbs that can assist indirectly in supporting other body systems, such as:

- Adrenal tonics (energy building and stress supporting), including Korean Ginseng, Licorice, Rehmannia and Rhodiola
- Immune supporting herbs including Andrographis, Cat's Claw, Echinacea, Hemidesmus

- Liver supporting herbs including Bupleurum, Dandelion, Globe Artichoke, Milk Thistle, Rosemary and Schizandra
- Antioxidant herbs such as Turmeric, which is also anti-inflammatory
- Nervine tonics (supporting the nervous system) including Lemon balm, Passionflower, Oats, St John's Wort, Skullcap and Verbena.

Herbal medicine is always best taken under the care and guidance of your healthcare practitioner. Always consult a registered, experienced naturopath or medical herbalist regarding advice and prescriptions for herbal medicine.

RELATIONSHIP SUPPORT DURING IVF

Men need to emotionally support their partner and reassure them at every step of the IVF journey. She needs to know and feel that the IVF journey is an equal priority for both of you and not something she has to deal with on her own.

When she's tired, feeling uncomfortable and bloated (due to the IVF procedure), devastated or angry and just needs to lie on the couch, the best thing you can do, rather than giving advice, is to make her a cup of (decaf!) tea, give her a hug and tell her you appreciate what she is doing for you, your family and your future.

Try to attend as many appointments as possible with her and show that you care by calling after she has her blood test and scan results to find out how it went and let her know that you are just as interested in the results as she is.

You need to invest a huge amount of energy into reassuring your partner that everything will be ok. It may be difficult to express your feelings as you don't want to say the wrong thing and upset your partner, but she will appreciate an open, honest conversation with you.

Share how you really feel about your fertility/IVF journey with your partner. Put aside the role of being the strong one and talk with your partner about how you are both feeling. Together, you can love and support each other.

STRESS SUPPORT FOR IVF AND MALE FERTILITY

Unfortunately, men don't always dodge stress either. If you are under stress, your hormones can be affected. Social and psychological stress can result in low testosterone and decreased sperm production in some men. Erectile dysfunction and premature ejaculation can also occur during stressful times or as a result of the chronic accumulation of stressful events.

> A meta-analysis of 57 studies with 29,914 participants found that psychological stress lowers sperm concentration and motility and increases the amount of abnormal forms of sperm.
>
> Li Y, Lin H, Li Y, et al. Association between socio-psycho-behavioural factors and male semen quality: systematic review and meta-analyses. Fertil Steril 2011; 95: 116-23.

Infertility and IVF are emotional and sensitive topics, particularly for men because our society tends to equate virility with masculinity. So, it is not surprising that men tend to bottle up their emotions.

Share your feelings with your partner. You are not immune to feelings of uncertainty, fear, disappointment and anxiousness. If you need more help, seek professional counselling. Most IVF clinics offer this service.

Naturopathic Stress Support

The good news is that naturopaths have at their disposal many stress supporting remedies such as:

- High-dose B vitamins - for adrenal and nervous system support
- Vitamin C – for adrenal support, immune health and anti-inflammatory benefits

- Minerals - such as magnesium, potassium and zinc, which are important for nervous system and adrenal health and for low mood/depression (magnesium is known as the original 'chill pill')
- Gamma-Amino butyric Acid (GABA) – an inhibitory neurotransmitter (brain calming chemical) which helps to relieve nervous tension, stress and mild anxiety, specifically for panic attacks and poor sleep associated with stress
- 5-hydroxytryptophan (5 HTP) – an effective nutritional supplement (amino acid) for anxiety, it assists in increasing levels of serotonin and dopamine, two important brain chemicals for mood health
- S-Adenosyl methionine (SAMe) – an amino acid indicated for low mood and depression
- Theanine – another amino acid with relaxing and mood enhancing properties
- Adrenal herbs such as Korean Ginseng, Licorice, Rehmannia, Rhodiola and Withania. Turmeric, a potent anti-inflammatory herb, has also been shown to increase serotonin and dopamine levels
- Flower essences e.g. 'Rescue Remedy', 'Emergency Essence' or Bailey Essence 'Shock and Trauma' (see next chapter)
- Meditation and visualisation techniques.

OTHER HOLISTIC THERAPIES FOR IVF SUPPORT AND MALE FERTILITY

TCM and Acupuncture

The benefits of Traditional Chinese Medicine (TCM), including acupuncture, on fertility is well documented, both in the classics of Chinese medicine and in research carried out worldwide.

Numerous researches show the effectiveness of TCM and acupuncture on overall sperm health. In particular, studies suggest that acupuncture can improve ejaculatory dysfunction, erectile dysfunction, sperm concentration, motility, forward-progressive motility, sperm vitality and total motion count. This may be achieved because acupuncture increases testosterone levels.

Acupuncture is also very effective at reducing stress levels.

A general treatment principle for male infertility is to reinforce the kidney, balance Yin and Yang, and tone and promote 'chi' (energy flow) and blood circulation.

Bioresonance

Bioresonance therapy is a biophysical technique based on concepts in acupuncture, homoeopathy and quantum physics. A machine such as a BICOM instrument picks up electromagnetic waves from the patient, modifies them and sends them back to improve the body's ability to regulate its own physiological processes, treating the whole person, not just the symptom.

The aim is to restore the body's self-healing, regulatory ability. Bioresonance therapy is a painless, effective therapy that is suitable complementary therapy for assisting not just with male reproductive health problems but also a host of other conditions including allergies and food intolerances, chronic fatigue, digestive problems (IBS, Crohn's disease), recurrent infections, joint and muscle pain.

Flower Essences

Flower essences can provide profound shifts on a mental, emotional and energetic level, yet they are gentle in action and don't have any side effects.

There are many flower essences which may assist men's mental and emotional state, but one to especially consider is Flannel Flower Essence, an Australian Bush Flower essence. It is particularly indicated for men because it helps develop gentleness and sensitivity they can share with their partner.

Homoeopathy

Homoeopathy is appropriate for all aspects of male reproductive health.

Remedies that a homoeopath may consider assisting with male infertility include Pulsatilla, Clematis, Rhododendron, Agnus castus, Aurum (gold) and Mercury. The latter two are members of the gold series in the periodic table of elements, which is known to have an affinity with the reproductive organs in both men and women.

Physical Therapies

Physical therapies may include massage, chiropractic care or osteopathy.

An important factor to consider is structural care. The tenth nerve and sacrum play an important role in controlling bowel, bladder and reproductive function. Therefore, problems with your skeletal system can have a significant impact on your nervous system and reproductive health.

For all of these modalities, it is recommended that you consult registered, experienced practitioners who have a special interest in fertility treatment and IVF support. For more information on all of these holistic therapies, please refer to Section 6 of *Making Babies: The Holistic IVF Diet Guide*.

Notes

BRINGING IT ALL TOGETHER

Here is a summary of the recommendations outlined in *The Diet Guide for Men.*

- Avoid/limit exposure to toxins and pollutants.
- Speak to your doctor about stopping or reducing drugs that may be negatively impacting sperm health.
- Keep your mobile phone out of your trouser pockets.
- Avoid tight-fitting underwear (including cycling pants), heated car seats and maintain a scrotal temperature of 34-36°C.
- Eat a healthy Mediterranean-style diet including plenty of high-quality protein, fruit, vegetables and healthy fats.
- Incorporate superfoods which provide important antioxidant support to protect sperm health.
- Avoid caffeine and limit alcohol.
- Lose excess weight.
- Stop smoking.
- Take specific supplements and herbs recommended by your naturopath.
- Exercise in moderation, although avoid/limit cycling.
- Get enough/adequate sleep.
- Look after/nourish your relationship and communicate with your partner.
- Reduce stress – practise stress reduction techniques and consider counselling.

By following the recommendations in this book that are relevant for you, you will improve your sperm health and in turn, give you and your partner the best chance of achieving your ultimate goal - a healthy pregnancy and healthy baby.

Glossary

Acupuncture – A treatment used in traditional Chinese medicine. Fine needles are inserted into specific points of the body to help promote and balance the body's system.

Amenorrhoea - The absence of menstruation.

Amino acid – Building blocks of the body which are different forms of protein.

Androgens - Male hormones produced by the adrenal gland that are sometimes elevated in women with PCOS, causing fertility problems.

Anovulation - Lack of ovulation that can occur with or without menstruation.

Antibodies - Substances made by males and females that attack foreign matter and help prevent infection; may also cause infertility in certain cases.

Anti-Mullerian hormone – Thought to be a useful hormone marker for predicting ovarian reserve, ovarian ageing, ovarian dysfunction and ovarian responsiveness.

Antioxidant – A substance that inhibits the destructive effect of free radicals that cause oxidative damage. These highly reactive chemicals attack molecules and can damage egg and sperm.

Antisperm antibodies – Produced by the body's immune system, they cause sperm to bunch together, thus affecting their ability to reach and fertilise an egg.

Asherman's syndrome - A condition where the uterine walls adhere to one another, usually caused by uterine inflammation (usually a complication of endometriosis).

Assisted Reproductive Technologies (ART) - Fertility treatments that include the handling of both the egg and the sperm such as IUI, IVF, GIFT and ZIFT.

Basal Body Temperature (BBT) - Temperature that is taken first thing in the morning after waking and that rises and falls due to changes in hormone levels during the menstrual cycle.

Bicornuate uterus - An abnormality in the structure of the uterus that can sometimes be fixed with surgery; can cause problems with fertility.

BMI (Body Mass Index) - is a height versus weight calculation of body fat and is a useful tool to calculate your optimal weight.

Candidiasis/candida overgrowth - An infection sometimes found in the vagina that is caused by a fungus and can cause burning, itching and discomfort.

Cervical mucus - Mucus produced by the cervix that changes consistency during a woman's monthly cycle.

Cervical smear - A cellular sample that is extracted from the cervix and examined for cancer or other abnormalities.

Cervix - A one-inch-long canal located above the vagina at the lower end of the uterus through which blood passes during menstruation, sperm travels into to reach the fallopian tubes, and the baby passes through during labour.

Cervix, incompetent - The cervix opens during pregnancy before the baby is developed and labour is ready to begin.

Chemical pregnancy - This accounts for most miscarriages as the egg implants itself but the embryo doesn't develop.

Chromosome - Structures that hold our genetic material.

Clinical pregnancy - A pregnancy that is confirmed with a clinical intervention like an ultrasound.

Clomiphene citrate - A medication that causes a surge of gonadotropins from the pituitary gland and stimulates ovulation to boost fertility.

Conception – The successful fertilisation of a woman's egg by a man's sperm.

Contraceptive pill – An oral medication for women used as a form of birth control.

Corpus luteum – The structure/tissue in which a follicle turns after ovulation. Its role is to produce hormones such as progesterone after ovulation and during pregnancy to boost implantation.

Cryptorchidism - A condition in which one or both testicles fail to move from the abdomen, where they develop before birth, down into the scrotum. Also known as undescended testicles.

Cycle - A round of fertility treatment that takes about a month between start and completion.

Cyst - A sac surrounded by a membrane; may or may not cause health problems.

Detox – Removing or clearing out toxins in the body, thereby preventing disease.

Dilation and Curettage (D&C) - A procedure to dilate the cervix and scrape away the uterine lining.

DHEA (Dihydroepiandrosterone) - A weak male hormone produced by the adrenal gland in some women that, in high doses, can cause excess hair growth and other symptoms.

Donor egg - Eggs donated by healthy young women that can be implanted in infertile women to increase the chances of pregnancy.

Donor embryo transfer - Donor egg and/or donor sperm are transferred to a woman's uterus during IVF to help her get pregnant

Donor sperm – Sperm donated by men who are screened for illnesses, ethnicity, build and other characteristics, and then usually frozen and held for six months or more before use in artificial insemination or ART.

Ectopic pregnancy - This occurs when a fertilised egg implants in a woman's body outside of the uterus, causing severe complications before it is terminated.

Egg - Female reproductive cell produced by the ovary, is fertilised by sperm during reproduction (also called oocyte or ovum).

Egg retrieval - Use of a thin needle to remove an unfertilised egg from the ovarian follicles to be fertilised by procedures such as IVF or ICSI (also called egg collection, egg pick-up or EPU).

Embryo - The early stage of the human foetus, between implantation and eight weeks of pregnancy.

Embryo transfer - During IVF, a patient's embryos are cultured in a laboratory until they are of a satisfactory grade. Placement of the fertilised egg (embryo) into the uterus is then performed using a catheter after IVF and other ART procedures.

Endocrinology - The study of hormones, glands, hormonal systems, and how they work together.

Endometriosis – A condition in which cells from the lining of the uterus (womb) grown outside the uterus. It often causes painful menstruation and infertility.

Endometrium - The lining of the uterus.

Endorphins - Substances in the body that induce feel-good and opiate-like feelings.

Essential fatty acids – Unsaturated fats that are essential for health. They are found in nuts, seeds, oily fish and some vegetables such as avocado.

Fallopian tube - Tubes connecting the ovaries to the uterus through which the egg is released during ovulation, where it waits to be fertilised by the sperm.

Fertility specialist - Doctors that focus on diagnosing and treating infertility such as a Reproductive Endocrinologist.

Fertilisation - The joining of egg and sperm which forms an embryo for pregnancy.

Foetus - Starting eight weeks after implantation, the embryo will be called a foetus until it is born.

Fibroid - A benign tumour made of muscle cells and other tissues found in the uterine wall (also called a myoma).

Follicle - The place in the ovary where a woman's egg grows and develops each month. During ovulation, the follicle releases the egg into the fallopian tube.

Follicle stimulating hormone (FSH) - A hormone from the pituitary gland that stimulates ovarian follicles to grow, and the production of sperm in the testes.

Follicular phase - The first phase of the menstrual cycle, starting with day 1 when menstrual bleeding begins and ovarian follicles start to develop.

Follicular fluid - Fluid that houses the egg inside the ovarian follicles.

Full Blood Count (FBC) - A blood test that measures red and white blood cells, haemoglobin and other factors to diagnose and assess potential disease.

Frozen Embryo Transfer (FET) – The replacement of embryos into the women's body that may have been previously frozen.

Gamete - A mature sex cell, the egg and the sperm.

Gamete intrafallopian transfer (GIFT) - A procedure where a female's eggs are extracted, mixed with sperm, and then placed in the fallopian tubes where fertilisation can occur.

Genetically modified (GM) foods – Foods where genes from another species are introduced into a particular plant to make them more resistant to pest, viruses or weed killers. In order to smuggle these new genes across the species barrier, scientists used infectious agents (viruses and bacteria). These antibiotic-resistant genes are used as genetic markers to allow the scientists to track the movements of these new genes once inserted.

Hirsutism - A condition that often occurs with PCOS where women have excess body and facial hair, due to high levels of androgens.

Hormone tests – Regular hormone checks for levels of hormones including FSH, LH, prolactin, oestradiol and progesterone. It is important to check fertility hormones are within the normal range to ensure ovulation and conception.

Hormone - Chemicals produced in one organ of the body that regulates the activities of other organs.

Human chorionic gonadotropin (HCG) - In early pregnancy this hormone helps to maintain progesterone levels; it is sometimes used to trigger ovulation.

Hydrocoele - Fluid accumulation in the scrotum.

Hyperprolactinemia - High amounts of prolactin in the blood that can suppress LH and FSH production, commonly resulting in amenorrhoea and anovulation, thereby fertility.

Hyperstimulation (Ovarian Hyperstimulation Syndrome - OHSS) - A serious complication that occurs with medically induced ovulation where the ovaries swell and mild to severe side effects may occur.

Hyperthyroidism - Excessive activity of the thyroid that can affect female ovulation and fertility.

Hypothalamus - The part of the brain that secretes GnRH, which enables the release of LH and FSH to stimulate the ovaries and testes.

Hypothalamic amenorrhoea - Defined as the absence stopping of a menstrual cycle. Typically very low levels of FSH, LH and oestrogen are found to contribute to amenorrhoea and infertility.

Hypothyroidism - The thyroid gland does not produce enough thyroid hormone, leading to a slow metabolism and fatigue, and impaired fertility.

Hysteroscopy - A procedure done using a hysteroscope, a thin, lighted tube that is inserted into the vagina to examine the cervix and inside of the uterus.

Immature sperm (germinal cell) - Sperm that is not fully mature and that have low motility.

Implantation - After fertilisation, the egg starts to embed into the uterine lining where it starts to develop as an embryo.

Impotence - A situation where a man cannot have erections or ejaculate semen.

Inhibin B - One of two hormones secreted by cells in the ovaries that inhibit the production of FSH by the pituitary gland.

In vitro fertilisation (IVF) - Meaning 'in glass', this assisted reproductive technology process involves inducing ovulation, extracting the egg from the ovary, and combining the egg with the sperm outside of the female's body for fertilisation.

Infertility - For women under 35, this means the inability to get pregnant or carry a pregnancy to term when trying to conceive one year, and for women over 35, infertility is the inability to get pregnant or carry a pregnancy to term when trying to conceive for six months.

Injectables - Fertility medications (usually ovulation induction medications) that are injected.

Insemination - The introduction of sperm into a woman's body for fertilisation.

Intracytoplasmic sperm injection (ICSI) - The injection of a single sperm into an egg, usually used with IVF.

Intrauterine insemination (IUI) - Sperm are collected and washed to prepare for insemination directly into a woman's uterus with a catheter and syringe.

Karyotyping - A test analysing chromosomes for potential genetic abnormalities.

Laparoscopy - A procedure to inspect the pelvis, ovaries, uterus and fallopian tubes using a telescopic instrument that is inserted into a small incision in the abdomen.

Luteinizing hormone (LH) - A hormone that stimulates the ovary to release an egg during ovulation, and also stimulates testosterone production in males.

LH surge - A surge of LH followed by the release of an egg from a follicle in the ovaries.

Luteal phase – The second half of the menstrual cycle, usually lasting 14 days, which starts after ovulation when the corpus luteum secretes large amounts of progesterone and ends with the beginning of the menstrual flow (a period) or pregnancy.

Luteal phase defect (or deficiency) (LPD) - Often due to a short luteal phase, the uterus will not be able to sustain a pregnancy due to abnormal hormone levels. May cause recurrent miscarriages.

Menorrhagia - Very heavy menstrual flow, or menses that lasts longer than normal.

Menstruation - Monthly cycle of bleeding where the uterine lining is shed after a woman fails to achieve pregnancy (also called menses, menstrual cycle).

Miscarriage – The natural loss of a pregnancy occurring any time between conception and 24 weeks of pregnancy. Also referred to as spontaneous abortion, it is the most common complication of early pregnancy.

Nutriceutical - A specially treated food, vitamin, mineral or herb that you eat or drink to improve your health.

Oestrogen - A female sex hormone that stimulates the development of female sex characteristics.

Oestradiol – The strongest naturally occurring form of oestrogen.

Oocyte - The female sex cell that is produced in the ovaries (also see egg, ovum, gamete).

Oocyte retrieval - When a needle is inserted into the ovarian follicles to extract eggs during surgery.

Ovarian failure - A situation where levels of FSH in the blood are elevated, usually indicating a lack of ovarian response to FSH stimulation.

Ovary/Ovaries - Female sex glands that produce eggs (ova) and female hormones (estrogen and progesterone) within the pelvis.

Ovulation - When the ovary releases a mature egg from an ovarian follicle in the middle of the menstrual cycle, often around day 14.

Ovulation induction – Stimulation of the ovaries by fertility drugs to encourage the development of multiple follicles and therefore multiple eggs.

Pelvic inflammatory disease (PID) - Infection within the pelvis that can cause fever, pain and possibly infertility and may lead to the development of scar tissue and/or tubal problems.

Peri-menopause – The time in a woman's life just before menopause when her body starts making less oestrogen and progesterone and her chances of becoming pregnant are reduced.

Phytoestrogens – Plant hormones that exert weak oestrogenic activity.

Pituitary gland - A gland located at the base of the brain known as the 'master gland of the endocrine system' that releases and regulates the body's hormones.

Placenta - This organ connects the foetus to the uterus via the umbilical cord, providing nutrients and oxygen for development.

Polycystic Ovarian Syndrome (PCOS) - A hormonal imbalance linked to infrequent ovulation that may include symptoms like menstrual problems, weight gain, pain, infertility, and hair/skin problems. It can prevent the normal growth of the egg follicles, causing multiple small cysts to form resulting in enlargement of the ovaries.

Premature ovarian failure (POF) - A syndrome associated with high levels of FSH and LH and low levels of estrogen, often causing menstruation to end before age 40.

Primary Infertility - Infertility in couples that have never had a successful pregnancy or in couples that have gotten pregnant but never had a live birth.

Progesterone - The corpus luteum in the ovary produces this hormone that prepares the uterus for implantation of the fertilised egg. It prepares the body for pregnancy after ovulation. It is vital in maintaining a pregnancy, particularly in the early stages, and in promoting development of mammary glands.

Prolactin - A hormone that helps women make breast milk after childbirth. Abnormal levels can hinder ovulation in women who are not nursing, possibly causing infertility.

Recurrent miscarriage - Refers to two or more miscarriages, especially if they happen successively.

Reproductive Endocrinologist (RE) - Doctors trained in obstetrics and gynaecology who are board-certified in reproductive endocrinology - the study of fertility, glands and hormones.

Salpingoscopy – A procedure where an endoscope is inserted through the cervix for visual examination of the uterine tubes.

Secondary infertility - Infertility that occurs after a couple have had a successful pregnancy and/or live birth.

Semen – Also referred to as seminal fluid, is a liquid medium that carries the male's sperm outside of his body and protects and nourishes the sperm.

Semen analysis - Examination of semen under a microscope to assess sperm count, movement (motility), and the size and shape of the sperm.

Sex Hormone Binding Globulin (SHBG) – A protein produced by the liver that binds testosterone and oestrogen in blood. It has a greater affinity for testosterone.

Sperm - Male sex cell carried in semen that holds genetic information from the male (also called gamete). This fertilises the egg during conception.

Sperm maturation - Sperm takes 90 days to fully mature as they grow and attain better motility for fertilisation.

Sperm morphology - Refers to the size and shape of the sperm. Abnormal sperm morphology can indicate male factor infertility.

Sperm motility - Movement of sperm. Good motility is a sign of male fertility.

Stillbirth - The loss of a foetus between 20 weeks gestation and birth.

Testosterone - A male sex hormone necessary for the development of male secondary sex characteristics, sex drive and sperm development.

Thyroid – A gland found in the neck responsible for producing the active thyroid hormone T4 and T3, which play an important role in ovulation. An underactive or overactive thyroid gland can contribute to infertility.

Trans fats – Fats that are produced from the process of hydrogenation in food manufacturing.

Ultrasound - High-frequency sound waves used to monitor pregnancy and observe images of internal body parts to detect any abnormalities (also called sonogram).

Unexplained Infertility - When no reason or cause can be found for a couple's infertility problems.

Uterus - A muscular organ that contains protects and nourishes the embryo and foetus during pregnancy (also called womb).

Vaginal ultrasound - Placing a probe into the vagina and using sound waves to view the follicles, ovaries, eggs, foetus and other internal organs.

Varicocele - Varicose veins found in the scrotum that cause an abnormal flow of blood in the male genitalia and can sometimes lead to male infertility.

Xenoestrogens – Foreign oestrogens which are produced from the environment or from plastic and pesticide industries.

Zygote Intrafallopian Transfer (ZIFT) - An ART procedure where a fertilised egg is transferred into the fallopian tube one day after fertilisation.

Notes

Resources

Contact Jenny Blondel, Naturopath

For further information about naturopathic medicine and its role in fertility treatment, or clinic information contact Jenny Blondel at jennyblondel.com

Naturopathic associations

For further information about naturopathy, and to find a practitioner near you, contact:

Australian Traditional Medicine Society (ATMS): atms.com.au

Australian Natural Therapists Association (ANTA): australiannaturaltherapistsassociation.com.au

American Association of Naturopathic Physicians (AANP): naturopathic.org

American Naturopathic Medicine Association (ANMA): anma.org

General Council and Register of Naturopaths (GCRN) gcrn.org.uk

Naturopathic Nutrition Association (NNA): nna-uk.com

The Canadian Association of Naturopathic Doctors: cand.ca

NZ Society of Naturopaths: naturopath.org.nz

New Zealand Natural Medicine Association (NZNMA): nznma.com

These are just some examples of naturopathic associations. For other countries contact the association within your country of origin.

Flower Essences

Australian Bush Essences: ausflowers.com.au

Bach flower remedies: bachcentre.com

Bailey Flower Essences: baileyessences.com

High Speed Blenders

Thermomix: thermomix.vorwerk.com

Vitamix: vitamix.com

Nutribullet: nutribullet.com

Index

Printed and bound by CPI Group (UK) Ltd, Croydon, CR0 4YY
03/11/2026
02243771-0001